The Manager's Guide to Six Sigma in Healthcare

Practical Tips and Tools for Improvement

D1565757

Also available from ASQ Quality Press:

Nan: A Six Sigma Mystery
Robert Barry

Nan's Arsonist: A Six Sigma Mystery
Robert Barry

The Six Sigma Book for Healthcare: Improving Outcomes by Reducing Errors
Robert Barry, PhD, Amy Murcko, APRN, and Clifford Brubaker, PhD

Lean-Six Sigma for Healthcare: A Senior Leader Guide to Improving Cost and Throughput
Chip Caldwell, James Brexler, and Tom Gillem

The Six Sigma Journey from Art to Science
Larry Walters

Six Sigma for the Office: A Pocket Guide
Roderick A. Munro

Defining and Analyzing a Business Process: A Six Sigma Pocket Guide
Jeffrey N. Lowenthal

Customer Centered Six Sigma: Linking Customers, Process Improvement, and Financial Results
Earl Naumann and Steven H. Hoisington

Office Kaizen: Transforming Office Operations into a Strategic Competitive Advantage
William Lareau

Improving Healthcare with Control Charts: Basic and Advanced SPC Methods and Case Studies
Raymond G. Carey

Measuring Quality Improvement in Healthcare: A Guide to Statistical Process Control Applications
Raymond G. Carey, PhD and Robert C. Lloyd, PhD

To request a complimentary catalog of ASQ Quality Press publications, call 800-248-1946, or visit our Web site at http://qualitypress.asq.org.

The Manager's Guide to Six Sigma in Healthcare

Practical Tips and Tools for Improvement

Robert Barry
Amy C. Smith

ASQ Quality Press
Milwaukee, Wisconsin

American Society for Quality, Quality Press, Milwaukee 53203

© 2005 by ASQ

All rights reserved. Published 2005

Printed in the United States of America

12 11 10 09 08 07 06 05   5 4 3 2 1

Library of Congress Cataloging-in-Publication Data

Barry, Robert D., 1938–
    The manager's guide to Six Sigma in healthcare : practical tips and tools
for improvement / Robert Barry and Amy C. Smith.
      p. cm.
    Includes bibliographical references and index.
    ISBN 0-87389-651-3 (soft cover, perfect bind : alk. paper)
    1. Medical care—Quality control. 2. Health facilities—Quality control.
3. Health services administration. I. Smith, Amy C., 1964– II. Title.

RA399.A1B366 2005
362.1'068'5—dc22   2005004133

ISBN 0-87389-651-3

Publisher: William A. Tony
Acquisitions Editor: Annemieke Hytinen
Project Editor: Paul O'Mara
Production Administrator: Randall Benson

ASQ Mission: The American Society for Quality advances individual,
organizational, and community excellence worldwide through learning,
quality improvement, and knowledge exchange.

Attention Bookstores, Wholesalers, Schools, and Corporations: ASQ Quality
Press books, videotapes, audiotapes, and software are available at quantity
discounts with bulk purchases for business, educational, or instructional use.
For information, please contact ASQ Quality Press at 800-248-1946, or write to
ASQ Quality Press, P.O. Box 3005, Milwaukee, WI 53201-3005.

To place orders or to request a free copy of the ASQ Quality Press Publications
Catalog, including ASQ membership information, call 800-248-1946. Visit our
Web site at www.asq.org or http://qualitypress.asq.org.

 Printed on acid-free paper

Quality Press
600 N. Plankinton Avenue
Milwaukee, Wisconsin 53203
Call toll free 800-248-1946
Fax 414-272-1734
www.asq.org
http://qualitypress.asq.org
http://standardsgroup.asq.org
E-mail: authors@asq.org

AMERICAN SOCIETY
FOR QUALITY™

Contents

Six Sigma is a management method based on the use of meaningful internal data, quantitative targets, coherent objectives, and sustainable performance.

Patient Care   5

What does the patient want? What does the organization need to do in order to serve the patient population?

Medical care is required for populations of patients sharing a diagnosis. Then, medical care is required for each patient as an individual. The population deserves national standard protocols. The individual deserves individualized attention.

A bottleneck is the part of the system that has limited capacity, compared to demand; that cannot easily or economically be expanded; and that limits overall production in an important way. In multistep processes, effective production planning means getting upstream planning right so the bottleneck stays busy.

The service line manager identifies with a population of patients served in order to have the global perspective. The service line manager has financial responsibility or else no one will pay any attention to him or her.

Getting high utilization rates requires continual attention by expediters charged with clearing away encumbrances that arise spontaneously in any organization.

Attract nurses by adopting the management practices known to attract nurses like a magnet.

Training and retraining are essential to the attainment of high and consistent performance. Everybody needs training. Everybody needs retraining.

Posting tracking charts does wonders for self-improvement. It applies to physicians, technicians, laborers, individuals, and groups. And it's free!

Topic	Page

There are three rules for effective task design: make the task more likely to produce the right result than the wrong one, make it possible to detect error on the spot, and make it possible to correct any error on the spot.

Gates are points in the process that stop action until upstream conditions are validated. Gates block the propagation of error.

Buffers are waiting times built into processes just upstream of irreversible actions to provide time to take stock.

Six Sigma does not accept go/no-go system design, but rather insists on targeting the center of the target range.

Charts provide management information and self-management information. Charts are a key tool for organizational performance.

Six Sigma process improvement goes through specific stages: define the objective, measure the baseline, analyze the baseline, implement trials, and control the results to be certain that improvements abide. These are commonly stated as DMAIC.

Topic	Page

Preface

Every healthcare organization has a process improvement program. The Joint Commission[1] says so. There are several to choose from. We believe Six Sigma is a good choice, and here's why:

1. Six Sigma is for line managers because it's goal-, action-, and results-oriented.

2. Six Sigma is realistic, dealing with manual operations, verbal communications, and other practices that are prevalent in healthcare but no longer common in other fields.

3. Six Sigma makes good use of information on hand and does not require outlays for data takers or computer systems.

4. Six Sigma applies to the very things that senior management is concerned with: patient safety, patient care, and asset utilization.

5. Six Sigma promotes professionalism and harmony in the workplace.

---

1. Joint Commission on Accreditation of Healthcare Organizations, Chicago, often abbreviated to JCAHO.

6. Six Sigma principles can be learned readily by present employees and staff; there is no need to hire new people.

7. Six Sigma methods can and should be applied to stay away from problems, not just to solve problems after they happen.

8. Six Sigma conforms to all Joint Commission standards.

Senior healthcare managers have little or no authority over many important participants and yet have responsibility for getting results. To use the most obvious example, physicians are not usually employees of a hospital. A community hospital may deal with hundreds of physicians, all of whom are independent actors. Six Sigma proponents believe that enlightened self-interest can attain a unity of purpose, optimizing the whole system and all the participants in favor of the patient. No reorganization of the system is required.

The modern American payment system is predominantly payment-for-diagnosis and not fee-for-service. The import of this is to drive the care provider in the direction of better utilization of assets. That's a good idea, surely, but how to do it? Much of this Six Sigma book is devoted to explaining how to think about, how to understand, and how to improve asset utilization while attending to patient safety, patient service, and patient treatment. Those assets include the nursing staff, where the only hope for having enough nurses in the future is to figure out how to increase the productivity of the ones available.

Six Sigma is the culmination of a century of learning about production management. What has been learned includes how to design manual operations to prevent inadvertent error, how to get lots of people to work together, how to manage bottlenecks, how to measure what's being achieved without disrupting the work, how to make changes with ample prudence, and how to know whether changes hold up over time.

Six Sigma's name is shorthand for *six standard deviations,* meaning that errors would occur only 3.4 times per million. That's not per million paper clips, it's per million treatments or patients. So, if a 200-bed hospital stays full and turns every bed over twice a week, that comes to about 20,000 patients per year. Six Sigma sets the goal of having not more than one dissatisfied patient every 15 years. An outpatient service seeing 200 patients per day would set the goal of having not more than one dissatisfied patient every five years. Unrealistic? Maybe. Maybe not. This speaks only of matters that are controllable, not of the variability in patient response to treatment.

Six Sigma says, set a numerical goal. It doesn't have to be 3.4 per million, but why not pick an aggressive goal? That discourages halfway measures and temporizing, it tells the community to expect progress, and it tells the employees and management cadre that you support what they support . . . what they went into the field for in the first place.

A hot discussion topic these days is, what does Six Sigma cost? A fair question, surely. Mount Carmel Healthcare System, Columbus, Ohio, has a vigorous Six Sigma program[2] with 40 full-time employees doing nothing but Six Sigma projects. These employees are drawn from various ranks within the organization, given some formal training, and supervised by senior managers. Did Mount Carmel hire 40 additional employees? No. Did Mount Carmel not-fire 40 employees? No, and certainly not these 40, who are among the brightest and most energetic in the whole organization. Evidence for this is that they are now being promoted to management slots ahead of their peers. Taking any five of these and turning them loose on any topic would very likely yield positive results, even if the words *Six Sigma* had never been uttered in their presence. Six Sigma awareness gives them a good tool kit to augment their talents and improve their production. Mount Carmel has a Six Sigma consultant as it has consultants for other initiatives; Six Sigma is not the only thing going on at Mount Carmel or any other healthcare organization.

So, the cost of 40 Mount Carmel paychecks can be assigned to Six Sigma. Or, one can say that the total cost of Mount Carmel operations is whatever it was before, and 40 peoples'-worth of time has been put to Six Sigma rather than to something else.

The cost versus cost-assignment issue, which is familiar to every senior manager, works both ways. If these 40 people were not doing Six Sigma projects, would they be doing other favorable things? Surely the answer is yes. So the fine-tuned question may be put: does the Six Sigma method provide some incremental benefit,

---

2. Personal communication, Tammy Weidner, VP Six Sigma, Mount Carmel Healthcare System, May 2004.

a benefit due to Six Sigma *per se?* We believe that it does, because Six Sigma addresses the management points listed at the beginning of this Preface.

Six Sigma can be instituted by having a substantial number of dedicated people, as Mount Carmel has done, or Six Sigma can be instituted by having a small number of people trained in the specifics who then coach others who are doing their day-to-day jobs. Use of outside consultants beyond an initial training period is probably not the thing to do; better to inculcate Six Sigma thinking into the organization.

It is sometimes remarked that Six Sigma is effective when the Big Boss gives the word. The conspicuous case is Jack Welch, who when he was CEO for GE announced that from that day forward, every candidate for any management position in GE would have to have Six Sigma credentials. That's certainly one way to get attention to the matter!

But the same thing could be said about keep-off-the-grass campaigns; they are more apt to be paid heed if the Big Boss speaks up.

Our position is that while Big Boss support is fine, it's not necessary. Six Sigma can be applied by any level of management (it is, after all, a management method): by small groups, interacting groups, large groups, and whole organizations. It can start small and move cautiously, or it can start with Big Boss fanfare. Big Boss hostility would not augur well, but what Big Boss is against improvement in patient safety, patient care, and asset utilization?

Six Sigma does some good and no harm. As management comes to master Six Sigma essentials, more good is done. And then more good and more good, accumulating and going always in the right direction.

Doing things right is less work than doing things wrong and then fixing them. Makes better use of resources. Costs less, too.

The reader may have noticed that *cost reduction* is not on the list at the start of the Preface. That's because this is a book for senior managers, and while cost reduction is everybody's everyday job, senior management has the larger role of managing the balance sheet, which is to say, managing asset utilization. Junior management can't do much about asset utilization, so it's up to senior management to do it. Those assets are financial assets, physical assets, and professional personnel.

Six Sigma sounds like something from a statistics course. This book does not shy away from using analytic methods, but only to the extent that they give management insight. This is not a statistics book.

Leave the hexanomials to professional statisticians.

Acknowledgment

page xxi

Ac-cent-tchu-ate The Positive
Lyric by Johnny Mercer
Music by Harold Arlen
(c) 1944 (Renewed) HARWIN MUSIC CO.
All Rights Reserved

Introduction

Six Sigma is a management model that starts with the understanding that the organization can and must meet very high goals for effectiveness by acting on information already available within the organization.

Six Sigma reinforces current developments in healthcare management: evidence-based medicine, service line management, and magnet nursing.

Six Sigma fits the real healthcare world, dealing with manual tasks and the exceptional needs of patients.

Six Sigma says: Aim high. Use information that is already available. Select the best way to do each thing, and do it the same way every time. Track performance.

Six Sigma even has a theme song, written by Johnny Mercer and Harold Arlen in 1944. The first stanza is

> Ac-cent-tchu-ate The Positive
> Eliminate the negative,
> Latch on to the affirmative
> Don't mess with Mr. In-Between.[3]

This is a book for management. Managers are always pressed for time, so we will jump right into things. This book is written in

---

3. Used by permission. See References (Mercer 1944).

newspaper style, with a contents 'front page' pointing to
for each topic. Each topic starts with a checklist and fc
additional information in increasing detail. Jump arour
interests guide you.

American healthcare is a great success story. There ar
positives to latch on to. There are a few remaining negativ
inate. There are some in-betweens to preclude. In-betwee
ally halfway fixes and patches, temporizing and incremen
Management can only manage a small number of change
so make each change tell. Don't mess with Mr. In-Betwee

Healthcare is a service business, so this book treats the customer
service aspects of healthcare as well as the medical.

Nothing in this book is foreign to healthcare. We recommend
wider application of methods that already work in various parts of
healthcare and, indeed, in many cases were first invented in healthcare, some of which were adopted by and further developed by other
fields of endeavor over the years.

You'll see that much of Six Sigma is common sense. Some of it
uses quantitative methods, most of which are already familiar. Some
topics may be new to the reader, particularly finite capacity analysis.
It's worth knowing about.

This is a short book on purpose. Your time is precious.

Here we go!

1

Six Sigma Particulars

Six Sigma is a management method based on the use of meaningful internal data, quantitative targets, coherent objectives, and sustainable performance.

CHECKLIST

☑ Manage the process, get the results.

☑ Aim high.

☑ The people will respond.

MANAGEMENT

The starting point is this: outcomes can be determined by managing the process delivering those outcomes. Managing the processes requires timely data and predetermined responses to that timely data.

Manage the process, control the outcomes.

Since healthcare is always labor-short, the 'timely data' need to be information that is already available or is very easily determined. We refer here to patient data as well as operational measures covering resource utilization, responsiveness to patient requests, internal

1

response times, and a range of other data. Each datum is almost always a very simple item, but one that has something to do with satisfying the organization's objectives.

Six Sigma does not use incrementalism. Instead, very high targets are set and efforts applied to get there in one jump. This always starts with taking stock of the present baseline so that there is a solid understanding of the current situation before something new is launched, even on a trial basis. When the baseline is in hand, there are well-established design tools for tasks and systems so that trustworthy improvements will be put in place, improvements that can be tracked and sustained over time.

While Six Sigma can be applied to individual departments, Six Sigma works particularly well when it is applied top-down. That's because policies and practices need to be consistent among interfacing organizational units, providing a global optimization in favor of the patient, not local optimization in favor of the individual department.

Six Sigma requires a management attitude that exudes the expectation that high standards of performance will be attained. People respond to what management communicates by thought, word, and deed. That is what top management contributes, in healthcare as in any organization.

HISTORY

Motorola invented the name *Six Sigma* about 20 years ago when that company decided to give its customers products that were twice as good as the customer expected. Customers had come to expect one failed item out of a thousand; on a normal distribution that corresponds to three standard deviations, which is commonly stated as *three sigma*. Well, if the customer expects three sigma performance, how about six? Instead of one failure out of a thousand, how about 3.4 failures per million?[1] That's a steep change in performance. Motorola committed to it, top to bottom, and got there. Once there, Motorola set even higher goals and kept on improving processes, year by year.

---

1. The arithmetic is shown in Appendix B, page 213.

Motorola also set ambitious goals in reducing cycle time, which is the time required to convert raw materials into finished product. This makes better use of productive assets, which is certainly an issue in healthcare as well.

Doing things right the first time saves rework. That saves time. Saving time is key to improving the productivity of fixed and inflexible assets. Purging slack from the system improves the productivity of fixed and inflexible assets. Managing the schedule and utilization of bottlenecks improves the productivity of fixed and inflexible assets. Indeed, the thrust of Six Sigma in healthcare is exactly this, to improve the productivity of fixed and inflexible assets while promoting patient safety and patient service.

Early Six Sigma adopters in healthcare include Mt. Carmel Healthcare System, Columbus, Ohio, which is part of the Trinity group, and Heritage Valley Healthcare System in suburban Pittsburgh. Many others in all parts of the country are now applying Six Sigma. Boca Raton Community Hospital, Florida, merits mention.

RANKS AND BELTS

As part of its dynamic flair, Six Sigma awards trained practitioners special recognition in the form of belts. The training of practitioners includes theory and emphasizes execution of projects:

1. A practitioner qualified to carry out Six Sigma projects is called a Green Belt.

2. A practitioner qualified to design and supervise Six Sigma projects is called a Black Belt.

3. A practitioner of advanced standing who is qualified to train others and to supervise large projects and multiple projects is called a Master Black Belt.

While these ranks are generally recognized and the qualifications for each generally agreed-upon, there is no national or standard definition of the qualifications for each of these ranks, although there are various efforts under way to establish such standards. There is no accreditation board for Six Sigma schools.

Some companies do their own internal training and some, for their own reasons, use titles different from these.

Nonstandard ranks, such as White Belt and Brown Belt, are sometimes seen. These have no agreed-upon meaning, although in general terms a White Belt is a novice and a Brown Belt has studied the theory but lacks practical experience.

Patient Care

2

Patients' Objectives

What does the patient want? What does the organization need to do in order to serve the patient population?

CHECKLIST

☑ Patients can reasonably expect outcomes consistent with national experience.

☑ Patients can reasonably expect attentive care.

☑ Patients can reasonably expect consideration of their time.

THE PATIENT'S DESIRES

What does the patient want?

- A cure
- Relief from distress
- A perfect baby
- No side effects

- Attentive care

- Consideration of their time

The immediate difficulty is that some of these things are beyond the state of the medical art. There are many medical conditions for which there is no known cure. No one knows how to assure a perfect baby for each new mother. Some patients react well to medication, some don't. There are limits to what we know, today. Maybe tomorrow or 10 years from now the medical community will know more, but at present, there are limits on what can be attained.

THE PATIENT'S OBJECTIVES

Since we don't know how to do all that each patient desires, we would do well to consider what objectives are reasonable for a patient to entertain, so that we can address those. Let's restate the patient's desires into aggressive, yet attainable objectives.

- Outcomes consistent with national standards

- Attentive care

- Consideration of the patient's time

These differ from the first list only to the extent that things that are beyond the organization's control are admitted to be so. It is reasonable for a patient to expect a medical outcome consistent with the state of the medical art, and if that includes a cure, that's fine. If it does not include a cure because no one knows how to produce a cure for all patients every time for that particular medical condition, then the patient cannot rationally set an objective that says 'cure.'

The medical outcome includes some measure of uncertainty. This uncertainty abides even if the treatment itself is exactly in accordance with the best known practices. This is an *uncontrollable* variability. Further research may reduce this variability over time, but right now it is uncontrollable variability.

There is nothing management can do about uncontrollable variability other than observe it when it happens and perhaps take action based on the observation. Management cannot change uncontrollable variability.

What management *can* do is to reduce all the other sources of variability in the outcome, in the attentiveness of the care, and in consideration of the patient's time. Six Sigma works to reduce *controllable* variability.

3

Patient Populations

Medical care is required for populations of patients sharing a diagnosis.[1] Then, medical care is required for each patient as an individual. The population deserves national standard protocols. The individual deserves individualized attention.

CHECKLIST

☑ Urge the medical staff to select protocols consistent with national standards.

☑ Urge the medical staff to select standardized care plans (clinical pathways).

☑ Track patient progress.

☑ Track population outcomes; compare to national outcomes.

---

1. Note on vocabulary. We strive to be accessible to the lay reader, and we eschew acronyms. The healthcare lexicon is not perfected quite yet (JCAHO 2004), and so we beg the indulgence of readers who might wish to see 'DRG' (diagnosis-related group) where we have written 'diagnosis,' and 'practice guideline' where we have written 'protocol.' For readers who would have chosen still other words, we beg your indulgence, too. Please feel free to write your preferred word choices in the margin.

CARING FOR PATIENT POPULATIONS

Start by encouraging the medical staff to apply evidence-based medicine protocols.

> Evidence-based medicine is a methodology for evaluating the validity of research in clinical medicine and applying the results to the care of individual patients. Evidence is gathered through systematic review of the literature, and is critically appraised. The results are then integrated with physician/ patient decision making. (NYAM 2000)

There are journals and numerous Web sites supporting the application of evidence-based medicine in the United States, Canada, the United Kingdom, and elsewhere. One example dealing with cervical cancer appeared in the *Journal of the National Comprehensive Cancer Network* (JNCCN 2004). Evidence-based medicine is endorsed by the National Institutes for Health, the Agency for Healthcare Research and Quality, and virtually all medical organizations.

The effect of this movement is to establish national standard protocols. The executive management question to its medical staff is, "Are we following the national standards?"

While it might seem that professionals would instinctively follow such national standards, there are well established reports (Weinberg 2003, 68) of groups of physicians who simply refuse to agree on what protocols to follow, inconvenient evidence simply being disregarded. In such cases, executive management has a simple but perhaps difficult policy decision to declare. Physicians are to follow the national standards or lose medical staff privileges. Following national standards is more defensible than not doing so, and that alone would appear to be a sufficient reason to encourage national standards.

It is not just lay administrators who find frustration here. Chief medical officers have commented to the authors that they themselves find it frustrating that individual physicians resist using the preferred protocols, always for some sufficient reason, at least a reason sufficient unto that physician.

Later in this book, the more general issue of overcoming local optima will be addressed (see page 83). Here, the *local optimum* is the individual physician optimizing on his/her own individual interests rather than the interests of the organization as a whole. That's perfectly natural, and fortunately there are ways to overcome, or at least reduce, such local optimization.

It is to be noted that this is not a new topic, and many methods from jawboning to financial incentives have been applied to encourage physicians to converge on agreed-upon protocols. Perhaps Six Sigma can provide a final nudge.

GETTING VOLUNTARY COOPERATION FROM PHYSICIANS

This method works with all kinds of people and groups, and it is a painless method for getting voluntary cooperation. Since there is little or nothing in the way of authority that can be applied to physicians, voluntary cooperation is about the only hope.

Six Sigma features graphical presentation of facts. When those facts have to do with the performance of individuals and groups, very often the result is that performance improves. Chief medical officers have told the authors that this applies in particular to physicians, who are competitive by nature. If score is being kept, they want to win.

Consider how this can be applied to attain high conformance to standard protocols, voluntarily:

1. The medical staff is asked to identify the preferred protocol for each diagnosis.

2. The results are tallied and circulated.

3. The medical staff is asked to reconsider their prior input.

4. This is repeated three times.

5. The final list, preferred protocols, is issued for information, no obligation implied.

6. Periodically, charts are issued showing conformance. Names are not shown; each physician has a secret code that is shown instead (see Figure 3.1).

7. Over time, physicians adopt the preferred protocol in order to improve their individual scores on the charts.

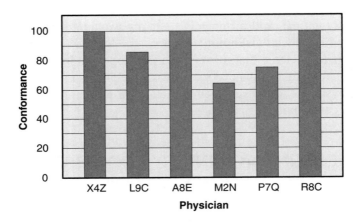

Figure 3.1   Use of preferred protocol.

Figure 3.1 is a chart showing conformance. Note that secret codes identify each participant. The code is known only to the physician and the data administrator, not to others.

In our example in Figure 3.1, perhaps physician M2N will reflect on the merits of the preferred protocol.

This is a painless method of urging compliance. If it doesn't work for every physician, perhaps it will work for enough physicians so that the hard-core holdouts will be sufficiently few and the institution can consider other measures.

APPLYING NATIONAL STANDARD PROTOCOLS TO EACH PATIENT

Standard protocol is covered in more depth in the next chapter. In brief: the physician is aware that patient populations include uncontrollable variability, and therefore the outcome is not preordained for any one patient. Tracking the patient's response to treatment is a necessary part of the treatment. In addition, any one patient may have other complicating factors that the physician will take into account in specifying the care plan.

Benefit of Being in the Pack

There are practical reasons to conform to national standard protocols. For one, more money and effort are going into medical research now than ever before, billions and billions of dollars, all of which buttresses the evidence-based medicine movement. For another, medical device companies are spending millions on improvements to sensors, apparatus, and tools—all pointed at the evidence-based protocol market. Small groups of practitioners with nonstandard protocols simply can't keep up.

Patients vary in condition and in response to treatment. It is helpful to any physician if comparable cases have already been dealt with by others. The likelihood of that is greater if most physicians are following the same protocol. This provides a larger pool of experience to draw on.

Staying with the pack is the best strategy.

There is an additional argument in favor of staying with the pack—the Experience Curve. The Experience Curve is based on observation of many industries, showing that the effort required to get the same output goes down as experience goes up. That stands to reason. What's remarkable is that the rate of learning seems to be a universally applicable number—20 percent per doubling of experience. This is covered in Appendix C, page 217. The import of the Experience Curve is that pooling experience leads to a predictable improvement in resource utilization. This implies that fragmenting of experience slows down resource utilization improvement for everybody—another reason to stay with the pack.

Comparing Outcomes with Others

There are now state and national reports on healthcare outcomes down to the hospital and individual patient level, and these reports are put out to the public without much in the way of cautionary notices to the reader. Any institution scoring less than average is immediately on the defensive (and any institution scoring above average is going to do some crowing).

The difficulty is that statistical comparisons, local versus state or national, are almost always suspect because the local count is too small. Small count → big uncertainty. Suppose the national survival rate for a particular protocol is 98.6 percent, and suppose the local institution treated 25 such cases and had one mortality, meaning a survival rate of 96 percent (24 survive out of 25). That looks worse, but is it different?

A few minutes with a spreadsheet, using just the built-in functions,[2] gives the following analysis:

Given the national survival rate of 98.6 percent, what is the likelihood that a survival rate of 24 out of 25 will be observed? Calculation gives 25 percent. This means that every fourth hospital, each with 25 cases, would be expected to show one mortality. So the local showing of 24:25 seems reasonable, or at least not unreasonable, and the local performance is probably as good as the national performance.

Since only one mortality is involved, what happens to the calculations if one more or one less mortality had been observed locally? That is, given the national survival rate of 98.6 percent, what is the likelihood that a survival rate of 23, 24, or 25 would be observed out of a total count of 25 cases? Calculation gives 99.5 percent. That seems to say that the local outcome is in good conformance with the national experience.

So, while the local mortality rate is observed to be four percent or 40 per thousand, which looks to be much worse than the national mortality rate of 1.4 percent or 14 per thousand, analysis shows that this could just be chance variation.

If the point is to show that the local performance is as good as the national performance, then this analysis is helpful, and the small sample size actually provides cover for a wide range of possible outcomes.

However, if the point is to figure out why local performance is better or worse than national performance, then the small sample size works strongly against getting any useful information out of the statistics. Trying to isolate subfactors means comparing even smaller counts, and the uncertainties balloon. Statistical computer applications will grind out answers, but they are so uncertain as to be suspect, if not just plain worthless.

So, let's see what can be done.

---

2. See Appendix A, page 205 for common spreadsheet functions. These particular calculations apply the binomial distribution.

Tracking Population Outcomes

Since patients are treated one at a time, it is helpful to track performance in a way such that each patient's outcome contributes to understanding what's going on. Here is a procedure that is quite easy to apply and has the same foundation as the chi-square test and other such statistical methods. The justification for this method is given elsewhere (Barry 2002, 198; Mood 1950, 365). The supporting arithmetic is given in Appendix F, page 235; here we will just show the application using typical values consistent with the case just described, national survival rate 98.6 percent and local survival rate to date, 96 percent.

The survival rate ratio is 96 percent:98.6 percent   = 0.973.
The mortality rate ratio is four percent:1.4 percent = 2.66.

We will calculate a figure of merit and update it after each case by multiplying by the survival rate ratio if the patient survives and by the mortality rate ratio if the patient does not survive. To start with, we set the figure of merit to 1.000. We will get a result after each case, and we will learn something from each case. This provides useful information as quickly as possible. See Figure 3.2.

If the patient survives, multiply by 0.973. Repeat for every success. Since this is multiplying by a number less than one, the product gets

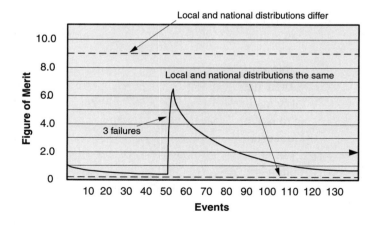

Figure 3.2 Sequential events.

smaller and smaller. Eventually, the figure of merit reaches the goal value, shown on the chart as 0.11.[3] Reaching the goal value proves, statistically, that the local and national survival rates are the same. Plot each point on the chart to show progress.

For each patient who does not survive, multiply by 2.66. This is a big factor, and the plotted point jumps up on the chart. If the figure of merit reaches 9.00,[4] then the local and the national survival rates are different.

For the sequence of patient treatments plotted in Figure 3.2, the figure of merit falls little by little as the first 50 cases succeed. Then there are three mortalities in a row. The plot shows that these three mortalities, while they would certainly cause some anxiety, do not prove that the local survival rate is different from the national rate. As long as the plotted points stay within the bounds of the upper and lower limits, the case is not yet proven in either direction.

This is covered more fully in Appendix F, page 235.

The point here is that there is a simple quantitative method based on sound statistical science that can be applied, case by case, to inform management on the consistency of local practice and national standards.

Note that no special effort is required to gather the inputs to this analysis because this analysis uses data that will already be known.

---

3. The goal value of 0.11 depends on the confidence intervals related to false negative and false positive outcomes, both of which are taken to be 90 percent. See Appendix F, page 235.

4. Ibid.

4

Patients As Individuals

Start with a standardized care plan for each patient. Track patient response. Intercede if the patient shows other than the expected response. Take charge of communications with the patient and family.

CHECKLIST

☑ Establish standardized care plans.

☑ Establish standardized patient information plans to match.

☑ Estimate the expected responses for patient data.

☑ Intervene when warranted, informed by the tracked patient data.

☑ Institutionalize maintenance of the care plans.

CONTROLLABLE VARIABILITY, UNCONTROLLABLE VARIABILITY

To get consistent outcomes, it is necessary to deal with variability in both of its forms, *controllable* and *uncontrollable*.

Deal with *controllable* variability by insisting that standardized care plans be implemented. That is to say, do things the same way every time.

Deal with *uncontrollable* variability, such as the differing responses of patients to the same medication, by tracking each patient's signs and intervening promptly if the patient's response is not within the expected ranges.

STANDARDIZED CARE PLANS

A care plan is a written plan based on data gathered during assessment which identifies care needs, describes the strategy for providing services to meet those needs, documents treatment goals and objectives, outlines the criteria for terminating specified interventions, and documents the progress in meeting goals and objectives. The format of the plan in some organizations may be guided by patient-specific policies and procedures, protocols, practice guidelines, clinical paths, care maps, or a combination thereof. The care plan may include care, treatment, habilitation, and rehabilitation. (JCAHO 2004)

Standardized care plans are not new. There has been a movement for some years to implement clinical pathways.[1] Some hospitals implemented them but let them go out of fashion over time. Based on anecdotes, it seems that where clinical pathways have been abandoned, it was because there was not enough nursing input into the pathways in the first place and/or there was no institutional discipline to encourage their consistent use or updating over time. These issues need to be dealt with up front by getting plenty of nursing management input into the detailing of the standardized care plans, insisting that admitting physicians start with the standard, making such modifications as may be necessary for particular patients, and, finally, by assigning responsibility within the organization for maintenance and upkeep of the standard plans over time.

---

1. Sometimes called critical pathways.

Pathways serve as an abbreviated description of the key events occurring in the care of a specific patient population. The events selected for inclusion in a pathway are thought to be significant contributors toward the achievement of targeted outcomes. (Wojner 2001, 92)

Clinical pathways are now widely published by leading institutions in the United States and elsewhere (Blancett 1998; Flarey 1998; Iowa 2004), so there is a good starting point for developing local standards.

The companion patient pathway needs to be developed at the same time and maintained by the same responsible group (see page 23).

Maintenance of Care Plans

Care plans need maintenance support. The nursing service would seem to be an appropriate place for this responsibility.

This is a line, not a staff, responsibility. Assigning care plan maintenance to a staff group is to invite desuetude.

Application of Care Plans

The physician starts with a preprinted (or on-screen) care plan matching the protocol, makes changes as necessary, and signs the order. The physician is typically standing at the nursing desk in the unit where the patient is being admitted. Therefore, the preprinted forms need to be inventoried at that location. If physicians also write such orders while in the emergency department, in their own offices, or elsewhere, forms need to be inventoried there, too, or made available to the physician via the computer network.

Bringing Six Sigma to Bear

To bring Six Sigma to bear, the care plan form needs to include the expected ranges of observable signs, such as temperature, alertness, blood oxygen, and so on, as may be significant for each protocol. These will be tracked, and deviations acted upon.

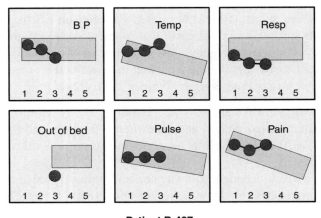

Patient B-487

Figure 4.1   Patient response tracking.

Clinical pathways are designed to cover about two-thirds of the target population.[2] They do not cover 100 percent of the population because the variability in the whole population is so great as to make any such planning meaningless.

Therefore, it is important that each patient's response to treatment be tracked and that attention be called when and where appropriate.

This constitutes monitoring for *uncontrollable variability*.

For instance, consider Figure 4.1. Bands, which are ranges of expected variation, are shown for each datum. The bands depict the response most patients will exhibit. Since some of the vital signs are expected to change over time, as in this example, those bands have a slope.

Patient B-487 is not seeing the expected fall in temperature and did not get up out of bed on day three. Simple tracking of the observables makes this manifest. The plotted points creeping out of the bands catch the eye.

These simple tracking charts facilitate and put a little urgency into figuring out what's going on with this patient.[3]

---

2. One standard deviation on each side of the mean, to be somewhat more precise.

3. For the difference between a tracking chart and a control chart, see
   Appendix A, page 205.

Note that all of this information was already available and recorded somewhere in the patient's medical record. Some hospitals make plots of temperature as a routine matter,[4] so this is merely an extension of a common practice. No new data are required. Some hospitals plot all vital signs, and some computerized medical record systems plot all vital signs. For these, no incremental effort is required at all, provided that the bands are planned-in for each standard care plan.

Which parameters to plot varies with the diagnosis and can be determined in advance as part of the pathway adaptation process. Since the pathway forms are to be preprinted, the bands for the plots can be preprinted, too. If the pathway is adapted for a particular patient to account for complications, then the anticipated course of events for each of the parameters can be adapted to suit. Indeed, if complications are present, then specific parameters may deserve additional highlighting.

There is no need to create the bands with high precision. The point is to help the professional staff spot unexpected trends and events at a glance.

Planning for and applying tracking charts organizes information for the concerned professional staff and goes in the direction of getting early attention to off-normal patient response. That's important, because it is known at the outset that about one-third of all patients will need some additional consideration.

Authorities in the field say that as many as 50 people who are involved in caring for a patient in an acute care hospital have legitimate reasons to access a patient's medical record (Abdelhak 2001, 56). Not all of these people are going to take the time to study the whole of the medical record, and yet all would surely benefit from having a snapshot of the patient's ongoing response to treatment. These tracking charts facilitate the use of the medical record by the whole range of users.

PATIENT PATHWAYS

Patient pathways are companions to clinical pathways and are structured information documents to be put in the hands of the patient

---

4. Factories commonly call their own tracking charts 'fever charts.'

and patient's family (NYU 2004). The patient pathway should inform the patient and family on what to expect not only during the hospital stay, but also after discharge. Common issues include: therapy, step-down care, diet, exercise, medication, smoking cessation, and follow-up care.

A common patient (customer) complaint is, "Nobody would ever tell me anything" (Gerteis 1993). This is the easiest complaint to forestall because the information is readily available. Why withhold it? Better to condition the patient and family to know what to expect.

Include the tracking plan and tracking charts. Update the patient pathway from time to time so that the patient and family will know how the patient is responding. If the patient's response is not standard, then this communication will lay groundwork for intervention if that becomes necessary.

Arming the patient and family with this information is to invite the patient and family to note and remark on any departure from the plan. This is favorable because it provides an extra feedback mechanism. For instance, if the patient is supposed to be gotten out of bed three times on day three, the patient and family will be counting.

With WebMD and other widely available sources of information these days, there should be no expectation of keeping the patient and family in the dark. Better to seize control of the communications channel to argue for the selected protocol and care plan.

5

Patient Protection

Protect patients from being harmed by any credible single failure.

CHECKLIST

☑ Identify the patient.

☑ Protect the patient from contamination.

☑ Provide defensive depth so that no single failure will harm a patient.

☑ Protect the patient from self-induced difficulties.

☑ Emphasize effectiveness over efficiency.

☑ Learn from every untoward event.

PATIENT IDENTIFICATION

Identifying conscious, competent, and cooperative patients isn't difficult, but then there are many who don't qualify on one or more of these counts.

The general rule is to identify each patient two different ways at every important point in the process. This is a useful guideline, but it puts the issue backwards. The need is to get a trustworthy identification of the patient, and among the ways of getting there is to find two independent identifiers. Machine-based systems don't need a second identifier provided that they have a trustworthy first identifier.

Let's do this in parts.

During the Care Episode

From the time the patient enters the hospital until the patient is discharged, it is necessary to identify the patient with a patient number. The patient number assures uniqueness, but it introduces the problem that people are not particularly adept at reading long numbers and getting them right. So the patient number needs to be machine-readable so that that particular human frailty is bypassed.

Bar codes are machine-readable and are now sometimes put on the patient's wristband. The difficulty with bar codes is that they are awkward to use at bedside and in the ambulance or in other unstructured circumstances because they require line-of-sight access. Furthermore, they are difficult to read from any distance because the laser needs to be shone directly onto the bar code. So bar codes do not constitute a general solution for patient identification even though bar codes are fine for many other healthcare applications.

Happily, the next generation is at hand. RFID,[1] which uses a tiny radio and computer chip about the size of a peppercorn altogether, does not require line of sight. The RFID tag, as it is called, can be buried in the patient's wristband.

RFID requires a reader, a radio, to query the tag. These range from little cards that insert into a pocket PC to larger sizes. The reader needs to communicate with a database to match up the number on the tag with a patient's name. In this way, it works exactly as a bar code reader does.

There are two families of RFID tags.

Passive tags do not have an energy source, they simply absorb some energy from the reader radio and send back the stored number.

---

1. Radio frequency identification (RFID). See Appendix E, page 231.

They have a range of several inches. Passive tags now cost about a quarter.

Active tags have a watch battery attached and have a range of several feet. Active tags cost a few dollars because of the cost of the battery.

Active tags, which can be read from the foot of the bed or from the doorway, are more likely to see wide service in healthcare. Passive tags, though, are promised by the major pharmaceutical companies for drug identification down to single-dose levels in the near future, just as bar code is applied today.

Passive tags are so small they can be hidden in the traditional wristband. Active tags are bigger because of the watch battery and weigh what the battery weighs. These may annoy the patient if added to the wristband, so they might better be used as an ankle band or name plaque. No line of sight is needed. Or, since a watch battery is included, why not give the patient a digital wristwatch that just happens to have an active RFID tag inside? Basic digital wristwatches are really cheap these days.

RFID is an enabling technology that augurs well for other aspects of healthcare. See Appendix E, page 231 for much more on RFID, including both recent and potential applications.

Linking to Prior Care Episodes

There may be information about a patient in the files, such as allergies to medicine, that should be brought to light. It would be advantageous if the link could be made using unimpeachable information. The best candidate is a biometric indicator such as a fingerprint, an eye scan, a thermal scan of the back of the hand,[2] or some other biomeasure. This is an active field of development because of the threat of terrorism.

Fingerprint sensors are cheap these days and widely used with PCs and handheld devices. These are contact devices, which is a disadvantage, and they require access to a finger, which may not always

---

2. This picks up the pattern of blood vessels under the skin, which seems to be distinct enough to identify the person. No physical contact is required.

be possible in a medical situation. Fingerprint devices also get more of the Big Brother reaction than other biomeasures.

Eye scanners do not require contact, since they are simply cameras. They do require a line of sight to the patient's eye, and they require that the eye be accessible.

Thermal back-of-the-hand scanners are also cameras so they do not require contact. They do require line of sight and access to a hand.

All of these require the cooperation of the patient to get the original data and to allow the information to be kept on file for this purpose.

Note that the application here is only to determine whether this patient has previously been treated by the same institution. There is no direct connection to the actual identity of the patient.

The simplest biomeasure is a photograph. Photographs do not discriminate as well as other biomeasures, but they are easy to create, easy to handle, and not threatening to most people. As a confirming means of identifying a patient, photos are reasonable. Author Smith has used photos, with the permission of each patient, to confirm identity of patients who make recurring visits to a cancer clinic. Wristbands aren't practical over an extended outpatient treatment program.

Actual Identity

Up to this point, there has been no need to know the name of the patient. To connect the patient with the patient's family and to connect the patient with a payer, the actual identity of the patient needs to be pinned down.

This is surpassingly difficult to do if the patient doesn't want to or cannot cooperate. We Americans refuse to carry national identity cards, and there are an enormous number of people who, for good reasons or bad, don't want to be identified.

Happily, a large portion of the population carries enough in the way of identification, such as a driver's license, that these patients are identified pretty readily.

That leaves a substantial number of patients who fall in between, those who would cooperate but for particular reasons cannot.

For instance, many hospital patients are residents in long-term care facilities. Most don't carry driver's licenses. The hospital can reach out to these care facilities and develop a consistent identification scheme and maybe get cooperation in building a library of biomeasures for the resident population.

Another example is sports teams. There are lots of trauma cases per season, and the players are likely to show up still in uniform without ID cards. The athletic department can create a library of biomeasures at the beginning of the season to facilitate identification.

Civic associations occasionally campaign to get kids fingerprinted as part of safety campaigns. These could be steered a little to include other biomeasures.

The institution can invite people to come to clinics for voluntary inclusion in the biomeasures library. The institution could add it to flu shot clinics. Small incentives like souvenir refrigerator magnets can be given to voluntary participants.

CONTAMINATION AND CROSS-CONTAMINATION

Carrying germs from one patient to another is to be avoided.

There are a number of encouraging reports of progress in reducing such problems. Here are two cited in just one issue of a multi-hospital quarterly newsletter (PRHI 2004, Q1).

Methicillin-resistant Staphylococcus aureus (MRSA). This was virtually eliminated in a large VA hospital by rigorous application of mask, gown, and glove changes.

Central line bloodstream infection. This was greatly reduced by using kits and checklists.

The favorable pattern here is to apply simple measures consistently. Find a right way to do a task, and do it that way every time. Give necessary support. Task design is taken up on page 147.

Getting lots of little things right requires the right working environment so that inadvertent errors are corrected and retraining applied if necessary, but no blame is laid. A blame-free environment is key to high attainment. See page 139.

PATIENT INADVERTENCE

Patients do not always act in their own best interest. Told to stay in bed, some get out of bed. Told to swallow pills, some fake it.

There are various sorts of bed alarms that conform to minimum-restraint rules, but there are other matters of concern, such as not swallowing pills, that don't have much technology support.

That is about to change for the better. RFID was cited above as an improvement over the classic bar code for identifying patients. RFID is also an enabling technology that will have far-reaching beneficial effects on patient safety. An RFID tag is a tiny radio plus a tiny computer. Add sensors for temperature, blood pressure, movement, and so on, to get an RFID-enabled low-cost miniature sensor that can track, record, and sound an alarm.

Some innovative companies are introducing products based on this concept. One is AugmenTech of Pittsburgh,[3] founded by Mark Friedman, PhD (Friedman 2004). These devices are expected to provide, at a low cost, information now lacking in acute care, long-term care, and even at-home self-care. Here are representative questions that may soon have answers:

- Is the patient out of bed?
- The patient fell. When? How hard?
- Did the patient drink the prescribed evening liquids?
- Has the patient moved enough to preclude pressure ulcers?
- Did the patient swallow the pills?
- Is the patient moving into a disallowed zone?
- Has the baby been dropped?

---

3. Author Barry is *pro bono* chair of the AugmenTech internal review board.

There are many more, so this list is meant only to indicate the range of future application of RFID as an enabling technology. See more on RFID in Appendix E, page 231.

DEFENSE IN DEPTH

When a new process or procedure is designed, it must be designed not only with patient safety as a goal, but with a depth of defense so that the patient is not even at risk. To state this more precisely, the design must be such that no inadvertent error at any stage ever puts the patient at risk.

The same applies to any mechanical or computer error, although in most healthcare situations, the risk of equipment failure is much less than the risk of inadvertent human error. This is not to dismiss equipment failure, but only to put things in some perspective.

An error-cognizant system has the following features:

- The possibility of inadvertent error is acknowledged.

- Errors are detected before harm is done.

- Single errors can do no harm to a patient, by design.

- Humans who make inadvertent errors are retrained, not blamed.

A small number of humans make malicious errors. Any such persons need to be identified and excluded. Defense in depth and the blame-free environment deal well with inadvertent error but not with malicious error. It is surpassingly difficult to design against malicious error.

System design and defense in depth are so important that they get their own treatment here on pages 125 and 129.

One thing to keep in mind is that patients and family often meddle with equipment within reach, perhaps innocently, but at great hazard. That's another input to the design. The equipment must tolerate such interference without putting the patient in jeopardy.

LEARNING FROM EXPERIENCE

We learn from experience by following these guidelines:

1. Be alert to nonattainment and negative outcomes.

2. Track.

3. Look for patterns and common elements.

4. Be cautious about jumping to conclusions; take time to understand the baseline.

5. Maintain the understanding that deficiencies are *system* deficiencies, not people deficiencies, and that remedies must be system remedies.

6. Be cautious about change. Test good ideas off-line and on a pilot basis. Get your negative thinkers to enunciate everything that might go wrong with the proposed change so that adjustments can be made beforehand.

7. If you make a change, make a big enough change to make a difference, with a strong preference for solving the matter once and for all.

8. If change is implemented, be sure to track long-term attainment to confirm that the improvement abides.

This method of thinking through and then managing change is an essential ingredient to Six Sigma and has its own acronym, DMAIC. See page 171.

Patient Service

6

Service Fundamentals

Patients want attentive care. All the lessons learned in other service industries are available for application to health-care. Think through the business issues, set standards, track performance. Encourage attainment.

CHECKLIST

- ☑ Identify the business issues of each aspect of patient service.
- ☑ Staff with service in mind.
- ☑ Set quantitative performance requirements.
- ☑ Track performance.

PATIENT FEEDBACK

Virtually all patient surveys show that patient complaints include the following:

1. Nobody would help me with my pain.

2. Nobody would tell me anything.

3. Nobody answered call bells.

4. We had to wait too long in the waiting room.

These show up even when patients' comments are generally favorable. Only one of these is medical, the pain issue. Physicians normally leave a standing order for each patient authorizing pain relief medication to be administered by the nursing staff. So, even this medical issue is in practice an issue of attention being paid, or not paid, to the patient. The patient wants attentive care.

We'll break this into four parts:

1. Being attentive.

2. Giving the patient information.

3. Responding in a timely manner.

4. Scheduling from the patient's perspective.

START AT THE DOOR

First impressions count; they count a lot. The patient's first impression starts at the door, or perhaps at the entrance to the parking lot. What's that impression going to be? What do others do?

Sam Walton thought about the impersonal nature of big-box stores, and he decided to put a greeter at the door, often a senior citizen, to push out a shopping cart and smile.

What's that smile worth in customer loyalty?

Sam Walton knew something about cost management, too, maybe more than anybody else who ever lived. Sam Walton made a trade-off, increased salary cost versus increased customer satisfaction.

Let's take Sam Walton's lessons to heart:

1. Customer service (patient service) has value to the customer (patient).

2. Customer service has a visible cost.

3. There is a trade-off between service level and cost.

4. Since the cost is tangible and the benefit intangible, there is a mighty temptation to save the cost and suffer the loss of benefit.

5. Management wisdom lies in figuring out how to do the trade-off and get the right answer.

Sometimes the visible cost can be offset. Sam Walton's greeters also check outgoing parcels just to make sure everything went through the checkout lanes.

But not always. Sometimes a cost is a cost.

How valuable is a first impression that conveys "somebody here cares about me?" Every service industry figures out how to value customer loyalty, as can a hospital, clinic, medical practice, or dentist. Then it's necessary to understand each aspect of the patient's experience with the service provider. That's usually done by semi-scientific means such as customer surveys. It's also possible to do this on a somewhat more scientific basis by doing experiments; fortunately, the experimenting can be done by observing what others in the field have tried, learning therefrom, and mimicking the winners. The others do the experiments, you get the benefit.

This only happens, though, if management makes the point of causing it to happen.

Should there be a greeter at the door? Or should the traditional Japanese hotel model be applied, where the reception staff who are not busy at any particular moment stand at the front door and bow deeply to each person coming in the door. Japanese department stores position employees at the top of the escalator on each floor to bow, too. (A smile works just as well and causes less stress on the lower back.)

A middle ground is to train all employees anywhere near the door to greet each person with a smile and an offer to help: a heartfelt offer to help. How much does that cost? What's the reward?

All of these things are probably already said to each new employee during orientation. How often are they repeated? How about a 10-minute video reminder? Wal-Mart does employee pep rallies every day. Guess why. For more discussion about employee training and retraining, see page 99.

BEING ATTENTIVE

Remind every employee that each patient and family member deserves 100 percent of the employee's attention for the brief time required by each interaction. There are stock phrases to be used (and others not to be used) to convey the right message. Say, "I'm sorry you had to wait," not "We're really busy today." No surprises here, but the fact is that employees need to be trained and retrained even in such basics. So does the medical staff.

It is also necessary that the employee in contact with the patient be someone who can deliver. Since most patient care is delivered by the nursing staff and nursing assistant staff, this is the place to start.

Maximize the number of patient encounters that include a nurse. Minimize the number of patient encounters that do not include a nurse.

This can be done by providing nurses, not nurse assistants, to deliver all patient care. Critical care units are frequently staffed 100 percent by nurses. Medical/surgical units are, in some hospitals, staffed 100 percent by nurses. That's fine.

However, it may not be practicable to staff all units 100 percent with nurses. Since the point here is to maximize the number of patient encounters that include a nurse, an alterative is to staff with 'care pairs' of one nurse and one nurse assistant, as is done in some hospitals today. Each patient interaction is with the nurse and the assistant. The two of them make beds together, serve meals together, give baths together, apply bandages together, examine the patient together, answer call bells together, and deliver medications together. The patient has someone, every time there is an interaction, who is competent to respond to issues. The nurse has an extra pair of eyes and hands to share the work, while keeping everything for which the nurse is responsible in plain sight. Nurse staffing is discussed further on page 95.

INFORMATION FLOW TO PATIENTS AND FAMILIES

Patient pathways, which are a standardized description in lay language of the care to be administered, should be provided. They follow the clinical pathways used by the physician and the nursing staff to plan the care but go further by sketching out the postdischarge care to be expected. That includes rehabilitation, diet, exercise, doctor's visits, smoking cessation, and other postdischarge care elements appropriate to each condition and adapted to the particular patient.

The patient pathway should be updated with patient-specific information as often as practicable so that progress can be followed. A daily update with latest vital signs and other observations is a step in the right direction. If the daily updates are shown as tracking charts with control bands, so much the better.

If the patient is in a disease management program, then the patient pathway should relate to the disease management plan (CMS 2004).

STANDARDS FOR RESPONSIVENESS

Many patient complaints start with the feeling that the care staff does not respond. One useful way to deal with this is to establish quantitative standards for performance and then to provide responsiveness consistent with that standard.

For instance, suppose an acute care hospital unit decides that the care staff should respond to routine call bell calls by going to the patient's bedside within five minutes from the time the patient hits the call button. Since occasionally there will be some true emergency elsewhere, it is impossible to promise that such a standard will always be met. Rather than using that as an excuse to make no commitment at all, it is useful to declare a policy that the five-minute goal will be met 95 percent of the time.

That allows some flexibility for true emergencies but does not vitiate the standard.

Given the standard, it follows that the unit will want to observe its conformance to the standard. The time of the call and the time of the response are probably logged already, so declaring such a policy does not call for additional data logging.

The simplest thing to do next is to make a tracking chart, post it, and watch how things go over time. Consider Figure 6.1.

There are about 25 points on the chart, five of which are above the five-minute objective, and three more of which are pretty close

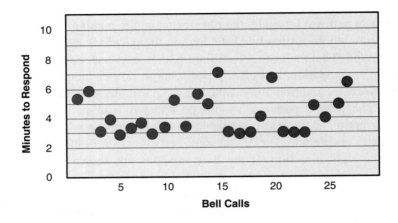

Figure 6.1   Patient service—time to respond to call bells.

to the line. Considering only the five that are clearly above the line, this shows that the objective is being met about 80 percent of the time, based on this set of data.

So, the *observed* service level is 80 percent. The *intended* service level is 95 percent. There is a shortfall.

A sample of 25 events is not enough to build a battleship on, and more data would help. A likely sequence of events is the following:

- The chart is posted along with a note reminding the caregivers of the 95 percent service level objective.

- More events are logged, and the service level would likely get better just because people want to score high in anything they do.

- After some additional time, the group will pause to discuss the following:

  - In meeting this objective, what other tasks are being given a lower priority?

  - Are we then creating problems somewhere else?

  - What other changes could be made that would free up resources for this task?

 – What additional resources do we need, if any, to get
 this service level up to 95 percent without jeopardizing
 other responsibilities?

 – Are we creating peaks and valleys in call bell activity
 over the shift? Are there other work sequences that would
 match demand to resources somewhat better?

 – If the objective were changed to, say, 7.5 minutes, what
 resources would that free up?

Note that the caregiving staff are not being asked to answer more
call bells during the shift, and therefore the total amount of work is
not changed. Dropping some other task to answer a call bell may
well introduce an inefficiency to the whole operation and some
increase in total overall effort, though.

So it would be interesting to observe what other tasks are being
interrupted by call bell responses. Are those tasks amenable to
being broken into subtasks to minimize rework if a call intervenes?
Can those other tasks be carried over to another hour during the shift
when call bell activity is lower?

Creative solutions may well come to the fore.

If the standard is set so tightly that no creative solution can possibly meet the target service level, then eventually management faces
a trade-off between service standards and resources. That's an appropriate management responsibility, one that is met in an informed
way if data are tracked.

While call bell response has been used here as an example
because it is an easy one to visualize, the same issues arise in any
service commitment to a patient.

COMMUNICATING SERVICE STANDARDS

Having and adhering to service standards is only part of the matter.

This started with the familiar patient complaint, "Nobody comes
when I hit the call button." So it is necessary to communicate to the
patient that there are standards, and that the patient can expect, as in
the example just discussed, that call bells will be answered within

five minutes, 95 percent of the time. The patient then has something specific to go by. The patient can keep a personal version of the tracking chart and so can the family.

The institution can publish the standards in brochures. If the standards are at least as good as the competition's, then the quantitative service objectives support an assertion that staffing is at the appropriate level, which is a favorable statement to be able to make these days.

7

Serving Impatient Patients

Patients who have immediate alternatives do not wait in queue. The only way to get their business is to have capacity to serve them, right now.

CHECKLIST

☑ Manage demand using standard business methods.

☑ Trade off occupancy versus turned-away patients.

☑ Scheduling some of the capacity increases the turn-away rate.

LONG-TERM CARE FACILITY EXAMPLE

Consider a typical long-term care facility, one of several in a community, of typical size. Suppose that promotion, pricing, location, and other factors are such that the average demand on this facility is 100 beds. That is to say that the combination of patients who are continuing as residents, minus discharges, plus people who want to move in, come to a total, on average, of 100 on any day.

That is not to say that the demand is exactly 100 every day. Indeed, the demand will vary quite a lot. Given largely fixed costs, the variability in demand is a serious management issue.

The demand very likely follows the Poisson distribution.[1] This distribution applies to things like the number of bank customers who show up on Thursdays during the lunch hour. It's a tiny fraction of all customers, perhaps 50 out of 10,000. It also applies to grocery store shoppers and patients needing a long-term care bed. Notice that while this is a probabilistic distribution, no probabilities are required. All that's required is the average occurrence level (number of shoppers who show up), which can be taken from experience. So it's easy to use.

The Poisson distribution has only one parameter, the average or mean value of the demand. In this case, that's stated to be 100 beds, on average. While the Poisson distribution has something of a bell-shaped characteristic, the spread of the distribution increases with the mean value. See Figure 7.1 for an illustration. The actual calculations can be done with standard spreadsheet functions. See Appendix D, page 223, for more information.

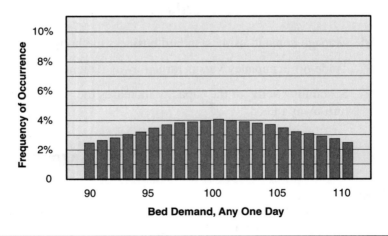

Figure 7.1 Daily demand for beds, Poisson model.

---

1. See Appendix A, page 205, for a refresher on statistics vocabulary.

The figure shows that the peak demand occurs when the demand is for exactly 100 beds, but that will only occur about once in 25 days (four percent of the time), and it is almost as likely that the demand on any day will be 95 or 105. Fifteen percent of the time, the demand will be greater than 110 beds, and 15 percent of the time the demand will be less than 90 beds.

As a practical matter, management has to set a maximum size for the facility. However large that maximum size, it limits the potential maximum revenue. In other words, if the upper tail of the demand curve is cut off, the average value will necessarily be somewhat lower. With a finite capacity and the upper tail of the demand curve cut off, the average *occupancy* can never be as great as the average *demand*.

Table 7.1 shows average occupancy for differing maximum facility size. These are all for the same average demand of 100 beds, given the Poisson distribution.

Note that even with a *capacity* of 120 beds, the mean *occupancy* is still not quite up to 100 beds.

Since the average occupancy is less than the 100-bed average demand, it stands to reason that some prospects are being turned away. Consider the 90-bed capacity case. How often is the demand higher than 90? Fifteen percent of the time. Fifteen percent of the potential business is being turned away. With a capacity of 120 beds, only one percent of the potential business is being turned away, but that takes more in the way of resources, and those extra beds will be empty part of the time.

Management faces a trade-off between potential revenue and resource commitment.

Table 7.1 100-bed average demand.

Capacity	Occupancy
90	85
100	92
110	97
120	99

Management has a certain amount of control over the magnitude of demand, because management can promote, adjust sticker prices, add amenities, take amenities away—all the usual things that any business can do. The difficulty is that management can't change strategy very often because much of demand depends on the public's perception of the image that management creates over time.

Business folklore has it that Mercedes-Benz, for many years, manufactured 80 percent of the demand for its cars. Why? Because Mercedes figured that creating an artificial shortage added to its image, and that image was more important than short-term revenue. Note that this means Mercedes was spending more promotional dollars than necessary to support its actual level of business. Mercedes was intentionally stimulating a greater demand than it intended to satisfy. That takes a lot of nerve and a rigid adherence to strategy.

On the other hand, the full-fare airlines have gone to great lengths to fill the last seat in every flight by selling the last few seats at a deep discount through online brokers and other gimmicks. This is not a different class of service; it's the same service at a knocked-down price. Since the cost to fly with empty seats is the same as the cost to fly with full seats, (even the flight attendant count is determined by the number of seats, not the number of passengers), there is a huge incentive for cash-hungry airlines to get a few bucks for that last seat. The difficulty is that this strategy works on image, too, in the opposite direction, breeding undying hostility among the full-fare passengers the airlines want to cover fixed costs. A death spiral ensues. The airlines who look like they are going to survive are closer to Mercedes-Benz in their strategy than to the full-fare airlines.

An interesting version of this, with a more positive flavor, is the practice of overbooking flights and promising, ahead of time, that any bumped passenger will be paid reparations in the form of cash, future flight coupons, and so on. In this case, what is being offered is not a flight, it's a package that includes the possibility of a flight plus the possibility of compensation. It's a different business. It also tends to concentrate demand on the most popular flight times because some passengers, and not just college students, angle for the reparations.

Carried to an extreme, though, the Mercedes strategy collapses. As Yogi Berra is said to have remarked about a New York restaurant,

"Nobody goes there anymore. It's too crowded." A turned-away customer will go elsewhere and may not come back. What is customer fidelity worth?

The Occupancy Distribution

It was asserted earlier that demand very likely follows the Poisson distribution. Capacity, however, does not. There is another distribution that has been developed that applies to exactly the capacity question. It's called the Erlang B distribution in honor of its inventor. See page 223 for more on Mr. Erlang and his distributions.

Erlang did his work a hundred years ago on behalf of the Copenhagen telephone company, back when adding one long distance circuit meant hanging another copper wire all the way from, say, Copenhagen to Elsinore. High fixed cost, variable demand. We'll see shortly that there is another distribution called Erlang C, which deals with a slightly different situation.

A 40-BED MEDICAL/SURGICAL HOSPITAL UNIT EXAMPLE

Consider a typical medical/surgical unit with 40 beds. Let's examine the same general problem, starting with a fixed capacity, high fixed cost, and low variable cost, at least for the last few beds. There is tremendous financial pressure to fill up every bed, every day, even while there is tremendous financial pressure to discharge patients as soon as they are fit to go.

With no flexibility in capacity, the only controllable factor is the demand. The hospital can increase demand by promotion, by adding medical services, and so on—all of which tend to act on a population of potential customers.

With a fixed capacity of 40 beds, let's suppose that the management target is to fill, on average, 38 beds. With the Poisson distribution governing the day-to-day demand, Table 7.2 shows what the average demand would have to be.

So, to get an occupancy of 38 beds on average, a demand for 50 beds would need to be stimulated, on average. But at this level of

Table 7.2 40-bed fixed capacity.

Demand	Occupancy	Turned away
40	35	12%
45	37	18%
50	38	25%

demand, 25 percent of the demand cannot be satisfied because all 40 beds will already be occupied 25 percent of the time. Another way of saying this is that 40 beds will be occupied sometimes, even though the average occupancy is 38, and indeed on some other days the actual occupancy will be below 38, perhaps 35 or 36. The fraction of days when the unit will have all 40 beds occupied and generating revenue? All 40 beds will be occupied 25 percent of the time.

Management, armed with this understanding, can assess the right level of stimulation to apply to increase or decrease incremental aggregate demand, weighing the revenue from higher occupancy against the image-impact of turning away an appreciable fraction of the total demand.

Pooling

One approach to dealing with finite capacity is to make pooling arrangements with some other provider of like capacity, such as another long-term care facility or another medical/surgical unit. This does not change aggregate demand, and it does not change average occupancy of the pooled units in the aggregate. This spreads the benefits around within the pool, but it changes both numerator and denominator consistently. There is no net benefit for the pool altogether. It might still be a good idea for other reasons.

Negotiated Demand

One common practice is to adjust demand a little by negotiating admission and discharge dates with patients, which does not change aggregate demand except at the margin, though it might have a beneficial impact on filling that last bed. This presumes that the patient, or a sufficient subset of patients, is amenable to being in queue at least for a modest period of time. (If all patients are flexible as to schedule, then this is the wrong chapter of the book to be reading, please proceed to the next chapter, page 51.)

The effect of scheduling a bed is to remove that bed from the capacity available for serving patients who are not amenable to scheduling and to increase the likelihood of having to turn away a prospective patient.

Suppose the same medical/surgical unit with 40 beds finds that five beds can be scheduled, leaving 35 available to serve the non-scheduled demand. Suppose further that management still has some ability to stimulate the nonscheduled demand to increase or decrease. Table 7.3 shows what happens.

Comparing these results with the nonscheduled case in Table 7.2, it is readily seen that the negatives (assuming turning people away to be a negative) are up for all levels of demand and the occupancy goes up appreciably only when the demand is not very high in the first place. If the demand is already high, there is no point in scheduling part of the beds; just let nature take its course.

Adding the scheduling of some beds may be good business practice for other reasons, and to the extent that beds can be scheduled, it may be possible to reduce other managed costs such as promotion costs, that reduce the demand for unscheduled beds. It would make for an interesting marketing trade-off study.

Note that it doesn't make any difference which beds are scheduled and which not. Only the aggregates figure into the analysis. Nor does it make any difference if some patients stay in the unit longer than others.

Table 7.3 40-bed fixed capacity, some scheduled beds.

Scheduled beds	Nonscheduled beds	Demand	Occupancy	Turned away
5	35	35	36	12%
5	35	40	37	20%
5	35	45	38	27%
5	35	50	38	34%

This is still Erlang B occupancy modeling, applied to the non-scheduled beds. See Appendix D, page 223, for more on Erlang modeling and how the actual calculations are done with spreadsheet functions.

8

Serving Patient Patients

Unscheduled patients who are willing to wait in queue for a reasonable period of time decide for themselves how long they are willing to wait.

CHECKLIST

☑ Queuing improves resource utilization.

☑ Queuing is a customer (patient) dissatisfier.

☑ Queuing requires some surge capacity.

PATIENT UNSCHEDULED PATIENTS

Emergency departments and some clinics serve patients who come in the door expecting to wait in queue for service. In some cases, once they come in the door, they are there for the duration because they have almost no ability to have a change of mind and go elsewhere. Others can pick up and leave when patience is exhausted.

That doesn't mean that these patients are going to be happily waiting for attention, and indeed they will likely be thinking dire thoughts every minute they are in queue. This can be mitigated by giving preliminary attention and by creating distractions, yet the fundamental issue is how much capacity needs to be provided for the level of demand.

A Model Emergency Department

Suppose a model emergency department treats all patients first-in, first-served; that the average treatment time per patient is 15 minutes; and that the general level of demand for the planning interval is known from comparable periods in the past (for example, Saturday nights with full moon). How many physicians should be on duty?

Suppose the traffic level, averaged over the period, would keep five doctors busy if the patients came in the door at just the right time so that every doctor is busy every minute and nobody has to wait at all. This is a demand level of five doctors-worth.

That doesn't happen, though, in real life. There is some fluctuation, and at some moments some of the doctors will be idle and at some moments there will be people waiting in queue.

Suppose there are five doctors on duty and that one doctor is idle for the first half-hour because the traffic starts out a little light. Then suppose that patients start coming in the door and that the average demand over the full period keeps all five doctors busy. Since the starting traffic was a little light, the average traffic over the rest of the period must be slightly higher than five doctors-worth to get the full-period average up, and five doctors cannot do more than five doctors-worth of work, so they will fall behind. There will be patients waiting at the end of the period. There is no catch-up capacity here, no surge capacity.

If the demand is for five doctors-worth of service over the period and there are six or seven doctors on duty, then there will be periods when several doctors are idle. Ah, but there is a surge capacity catch-up if, due to a temporary surge in traffic, the doctors get behind. There still will be periods when some patients have to wait for service.

It is possible to calculate the expected fraction of patients who have to wait at all, and it is possible to calculate how many of them have to wait longer than a "reasonable" period of time in queue. See Table 8.1.

Having five doctors on duty doesn't work for lack of surge capacity, as was discussed. Having six doctors on duty works pretty

Table 8.1 Emergency department, traffic is five doctors-worth.

Traffic, in doctors-worth	Doctors on duty	Fraction of patients who wait less than 30 minutes
5	5	Indeterminate
5	6	92%
5	7	99%

Table 8.2 Patients served within 30 minutes.

Traffic, in doctors-worth	Doctors on duty					
	4	**5**	**6**	**7**	**8**	**9**
3	93%	99%	100%	100%	100%	100%
4		92%	99%	100%	100%	100%
5			92%	99%	100%	100%
6				92%	100%	100%
7					92%	99%

well, with 92 percent of the patients being served within half an hour. Having seven doctors on duty works even better, with 99 percent of patients served in half an hour. The difficulty is obvious; revenue for five doctors is being generated and the cost of six or seven doctors is being borne.

The management issue may be stated thusly: is the business value of increased customer satisfaction, generated by seeing 99 percent rather than 92 percent of patients within half an hour, sufficiently high as to cover the cash cost of the additional physician being on duty during this period?

Table 8.2 is a more general table, covering more combinations of traffic and capacity.[1]

This table shows the interesting effect that providing one doctor beyond the nominal traffic level gives a service level of 90 percent or so, (patients seen within half an hour), and adding a second doctor

---

1. How to do the calculations will be taken up shortly.

beyond the nominal traffic level gives nearly 100 percent service level. This probably argues for one doctor beyond the nominal more than it argues for two, although the point here is that now an informed trade-off can be made by management.

This analysis is done using the Erlang C distribution. Erlang was with a telephone company, and one of the questions in those days, circa 1908, was how long customers would be willing to wait for a dial tone[2] or for an operator to say "Number please."[3] It's the same modeling problem, and Erlang was clever enough to figure out the arithmetic, which is related to the Poisson distribution but takes account of the queuing, too. For more specifics on Erlang distributions, see Appendix D, page 223.

The formal unit for counting traffic is not doctors-worth but *erlangs*. Telephone traffic and all other sorts of traffic are counted in erlangs, which is a unit recognized by the International Organization for Standardization (ISO). One erlang of traffic will keep one unit of capacity occupied for one unit of time.

PRIORITY QUEUES

Emergency departments have to deal with *emergencies* on a priority basis. Emergency departments often have an intermediate level, called *urgent,* which is below emergent but above standard. Emergency patients go to the front of the queue, urgent patients go next, and finally standard patients get a turn.

Since emergency patients do not wait at all, provided the number of doctors exceeds the number of emergency patients at any moment, emergency patients are not the ones who are waiting in queue. Nor are the urgent patients the ones waiting in queue. The ones doing the waiting in queue are the standard patients.

Therefore, Table 8.2 saying, for instance, that 92 percent of patients are being seen within 30 minutes should be restated to say that emergent and urgent patients go to the front of the line and that

---

2. Automatic dialing began in 1891 in Kansas City. It took a while to catch on.

3. This was the Copenhagen telephone company, so make that "Nummer, behage."

Table 8.3 Fraction of nonpriority patients waiting 30 minutes for care, given that eight percent of total population wait 30 minutes or more.

Fraction of patients who get priority	Fraction of nonpriority patients who wait 30 minutes or more
0%	8%
10%	9%
20%	10%
30%	11%
40%	13%
50%	16%
60%	20%
70%	27%
80%	40%

(some percentage of) standard patients are served within 30 minutes. What is that percentage?

It depends on the mix of traffic. Suppose a third of the total traffic is emergent and urgent traffic. Using the data in Table 8.2, some eight percent of *total* patients (100 percent to 92 percent) are in queue for more than 30 minutes. Assigning all that queuing to the ⅔ of patients who are standard patients means that, not eight percent, but rather 12 percent of standard patients are waiting for 30 minutes or more.

Table 8.3 shows how the mix of traffic drives the queue of standard patients.

So, as the fraction of total traffic that is priority traffic exceeds half, the queuing burden on nonpriority patients looks to be getting out of hand. No surprise here, and the quantification helps to inform management so that suitable staffing and planning decisions can be made.

SEGREGATING LOW-INTENSITY TRAFFIC

One alterative to adding doctors to improve queuing time is to segregate low-intensity traffic, taking this low-intensity traffic out of the population to be served. Low-intensity traffic would be patients who need some attention but do not need to see a fully qualified physician. Perhaps they need to have a bandage rewrapped or a ring cut off.

This has two immediate effects. One is to reduce the total traffic being seen by the emergency department doctors. The other is to raise the mix of priority traffic (by taking away only nonpriority traffic). The net effect can be figured out by following the analytic method used earlier with new parameters.

If one doctors-worth of low-intensity traffic is taken away and the number of doctors on duty kept the same, the queuing time goes down. However, somebody has to staff the low-intensity work and there is no increase in revenue, so there is a strong temptation to reduce the number of doctors by one. Let's look at the impact on queuing in Table 8.4.

If low-intensity traffic is taken away and the number of doctors stays the same, queuing goes down (see second row). That stands to reason. Then, if one doctor is taken away, queuing goes back up (see third row). That stands to reason, too. The net effect for this particular mix of traffic is to make things worse, if *worse* is taken to mean the higher fraction of nonpriority patients who are required to wait 30 minutes or more.

Meanwhile, the low-intensity care has to be staffed by suitable professionals. Management is free to define *low intensity* to suit itself, so this could be limited to medical matters that a nurse or a nurse-practitioner could deal with.

Now, what's the queuing situation in the low-intensity unit? If the low-intensity traffic is one doctors-worth and the capacity is one

Table 8.4 Impact on queuing with low-intensity traffic removed; nonpriority traffic reduced by one doctors-worth.

Priority traffic	Nonpriority traffic	Total traffic	Doctors on duty	Nonpriority patients in queue for 30 minutes
2	3	5	6	13%
2	2	4	6	2%
2	2	4	5	16%

unit, then the queuing time is indeterminate, which is to say it might be long because there is no surge capacity to recover if a surge in traffic follows a lull in traffic. If two practitioners are provided, then it is not likely that this is a winning game; the labor cost of the extra practitioner will overwhelm the labor savings that drove this stratagem in the first place.

Since this low-intensity traffic is, by definition, of low medical intensity, it may be useful to try payoff schemes such as those used by airlines: "Free visit if you have to wait in the low-intensity queue for more than 30 minutes." Or some other bounty. Given that most patients are not first-party payers, 'free service' is probably a less powerful bonus than some other item of value. Free T-shirt. Free eye exam. Free aspirin. Free WiFi. The point is to change the terms of engagement so that the patient's focus is not entirely on queuing time. Look for some patients to bunch themselves up to angle for that free T-shirt, though.

THE LAW OF STRATIFIED LABOR GRADES

Low-intensity patients might note at a particular moment that the queue is longer in the low-intensity unit than in the emergency department, so they jump back into that shorter line. While this might benefit those particular patients, the impact is to increase queuing in the emergency department for the next patients coming in (because traffic is up) while reducing queuing in the low-intensity unit (because traffic is down). The patient who jumped to the shorter queue gets quicker service, but the next high-intensity patient who comes in the door will be waiting longer.

Note that this self-switching only works in one direction. A high-intensity patient cannot benefit from switching to the low-intensity line because the skills there don't match the need.

Stratified labor grades *always* go in the direction of increasing the duty of the higher labor grades while reducing the duty of the lower labor grades, with a net negative impact on overall service.

Lower labor grades tend to be idle; higher labor grades tend to be overworked.

This *law of stratified labor grades* is valid for any circumstances where the work is not 100 percent predictable. In the matter being discussed here, the patient creates the variability by choosing which line to stand in. In other cases, such as nursing service staffing in medical/surgical care units, the variability arises when patients respond in unpredictable ways to treatment. The higher labor grades are the most flexible, so they wind up responding to the variability while lower labor grades stand idle, or at least less overworked.

The more labor grades, the higher the likelihood that the lowest grades will be idle.

Two layers might work, as with the low-intensity alternative to the full-treatment emergency department, coupled with a clever bonus plan to take the edge off queuing time in the low-intensity line. Three layers are not apt to work at all.

COMPUTER QUEUING MODELS

Erlang did his work long before computers existed, and today even desktop computers can do elaborate queuing models to give much more detail.

They also take more effort to set up, and they almost always require much more in the way of input.

Given that patient traffic itself is inherently unpredictable beyond general historical averages, the outputs of analysis are going to be inherently imprecise.

In short, fancy analysis doesn't provide much more management insight than 'simple' Erlang analysis. Indeed, fancy analysis often creates an illusion of precision not at all warranted by the quality of the input data. So, go easy on the computer modeling.

SEQUENCES AND BOTTLENECKS

The *traffic versus capacity* service-level analysis in this chapter has dealt with one-stage events such as a patient's encounter with an emergency department. In a later chapter, bottlenecks in multistage treatment processes will be addressed. See page 73.

To sum this topic up for the impatient reader, multistage processes need to be scheduled both ways from the bottleneck. The bottleneck has no surge capacity, by definition, and cannot catch up if it gets behind or is starved by a lull in patient traffic. So steps need to be taken to minimize the likelihood that the bottleneck ever hits a lull in traffic. It's a good chapter, worth the reading. It even has some Japanese words, with translations.

9

Serving Scheduled Patients

Scheduling services reduces capacity. Scheduling is for the benefit of the patient. Make sure the patient appreciates it by working on the total patient experience.

CHECKLIST

☑ Design the scheduled service to minimize capacity loss.

☑ Allow for surge capacity.

☑ Work on the totality of the patient experience.

CAPACITY IMPACT

Designing capacity to respond to the overall demand was considered in Chapter 8 on *unscheduled* care. The same general considerations apply to *scheduled* care, which is to say, for the care of patients whose conditions allow for selecting a treatment time within a time window.

Here's why the capacity impact of scheduling is negative. If patients are not scheduled but simply waiting in queue, then there is no productive time lost between patients; the doctor goes from one patient to the next until the entire queue goes dry. Doctor productivity is maximized.

Now consider what happens if patients are not in queue but show up on the quarter-hour. Suppose Doctor Jones treats the first patient in eight minutes. Doctor Jones then waits seven minutes until the next patient comes in. Doctor Jones can never make up those seven minutes of nonproductive time. Doctor Jones's productive capacity is reduced by seven minutes for the day.

Now consider what happens if two or three patients in a row happen to take longer than the mean time to be treated, resulting in a backup and causing downstream patients to be delayed. In setting up schedules in the first place, Dr. Jones had purposefully given up capacity to earn patient satisfaction, and now Dr. Jones must give up some more capacity to avoid losing satisfaction among those downstream patients being delayed. Dr. Jones needs to plan-in some time buffers to provide surge capacity, or catch-up capacity, for just these situations. So this is a second hit on productivity. Since the doctor cannot know ahead of time which patients will take the longer times, the only thing to do is to plan-in these catch-up time buffers into each day's schedule. Since on most days the aggregate of patients will be treated in the average time, then on most days the doctor will be idle for the aggregate number of minutes in those catch-up buffer periods.

So, the business strategy of scheduling patients to earn goodwill leads to doctor idle-time on the average day. That's a loss of productive capacity. Scheduling may well be the best business strategy. The only point here is that there is necessarily a capacity cost concomitant with this business strategy.

While the discussion here has been in terms of a doctor as the unit of production, the same discussion applies to any unit of production, such as an MRI unit, whose capacity may not be tied directly to the availability of a doctor.

REINFORCING THE STRATEGY AND RECOVERING SOME CAPACITY

Having made the business decision to schedule patient visits, here are steps to consider to reinforce the goodwill earned by the scheduling in the first place and to recover some of the capacity without eroding that precious goodwill:

1. Work on the total patient experience.

2. Reduce variability in treatment time.

3. Schedule patients in small flights.

The Total Experience

Given the business decision to provide scheduled service, solely for the benefit of the patient, then it is prudent to address all aspects of the patient's encounter with the service event.

Minimize the Demand on the Patient's Time

To reduce the time the patient will spend at the service location on treatment day, see how many things can be taken care of on a prior day and see what controllable sources of variability can be taken into hand ahead of time. Questions to ask include:

- How is the patient going to get to the service location? Are there time windows on that transportation? How reliable is that transportation?

- How is the patient going to be identified on the day of treatment? Can identification be assured ahead of time with a thumb print or a photo?

- Can the patient be examined ahead of time?

- Can the patient be oriented ahead of time?

Explain to the patient and family that these things are being dealt with early for the very reason of reducing the patient's time on treatment day(s). It's favorable. Take credit.

Give Schedule Specifics

Give the patient and family specific instructions that convey that the schedule is really the schedule. "Be here at 8:45 for sign-in. You'll be shown to the treatment room by 9:00. Doctor Jones will see you between 9:00 and 9:45. You'll be finished before 10:00." More information, and particularly more specific information, works, reinforcing the sales message that the patient's time is regarded as precious.

Track and Show

Keep a tracking chart in plain sight showing success in meeting the see-doctor times and the ready-to-leave times. Show the 90 percent and 95 percent success lines. The tracking chart is a built-in defense for that one day when things go haywire and some few patients are held up. The 95 percent line will be impinged about one day a month (one time in 20), so the need for a defense will always be necessary. Still, that's better than having to listen to complaints every day!

Schedule Small Flights

Scheduling each patient into a distinct time block gives up too much productivity. Here's why.

Suppose that experience shows that the doctor spends an average of 10 minutes with office patients, with a standard deviation in the contact time of five minutes. If patients were scheduled 20 minutes apart (mean plus two standard deviations), 95 percent of the time each patient would be completed within the 20-minute time block, and only one subsequent patient out of 20 would be delayed at all. That would be very good patient service, but at a substantial cost . . . 20 minutes being allowed to provide a service that on average only takes 10 minutes to perform.

On the other hand, if the patients are scheduled 10 minutes apart, half will be delayed and a quarter delayed substantially. So that would defeat the whole purpose of scheduling patients in the first place (customer satisfaction).

Here's a way of delivering what was promised while getting reasonable productivity. Schedule the patients in small *flights*, by which is meant in small groups.

Suppose a flight of two patients is booked for 8:00 AM and both patients are prepped in parallel. The doctor sees one patient and then goes immediately to the next patient. If both patients are average, then the doctor will be done at 8:20 AM. If some time is allowed so that, with 95% confidence, the next pair of patients can be started with no delay, at what time should those next patients be booked? It turns out that they can be booked for 8:35 AM. If each patient had been booked separately, one would have been at 8:00 AM, the second at 8:20 AM, and the third at 8:40 AM. So, we regained five minutes out of 40, which is 16%, meaning the doctor can see 16% more patients over the day, while giving each 95% confidence of being started on time.

Here's the arithmetic to figure the new starting time for patients 3 and 4 to be at 8:35 AM. The average times just add together. The variances add, which means that the standard deviations[1] add like the sides of triangles, square root of the sum of the squares. It stands to reason that sometimes one patient will take longer and the next one shorter, so the sum of the two together are a little less spread out in time.

Note that while both of the first two patients are started at 8:00 AM, only one is seen by the doctor at that moment; the other waits until the doctor is through with the first patient, an average wait of 10 minutes. That is probably not unreasonable, because most patients, having been prepped, would not be irate over a wait of 10 minutes.

But suppose we start a flight of three patients at 8:00 AM. Patient 2 would wait 10 minutes and patient 3 20 minutes on most days. Twenty minutes would be tolerable, probably. The doctor's productivity would be up, because the next flight of three patients could be booked for 8:50 AM, another gain of five minutes.

If we book flights of four, five, and more patients, we can continue to increase revenue, while paying for it by making more and more patients annoyed by longer and longer waits. Following are two figures to show the effects. The charts consider the four-hour time block between 8:00 AM and noon. Figure 9.1 shows the number of patients who will out by noon. The lines would be a little smoother if patients were counted if they were released by five or 10

---

1. The *standard deviation* is defined as the square root of the variance. See the Special Vocabulary refresher section, Appendix A, page 205. The standard deviation can be computed with standard spreadsheet functions, page 210.

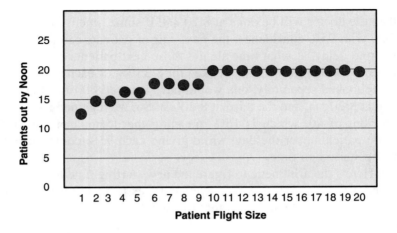

Figure 9.1 Patient flight-size planning.

minutes after noon, but to keep things simple, only those who are released by noon are counted here.

Recall that the average patient time is 10 minutes, and there are 24 10-minute blocks in the four hours between 8:00 AM and noon, so the maximum number of 10-minute patient encounters is 24. Allowing for some variability and using the mean time of 10 minutes and the standard deviation of five minutes, 20 is about the largest number of patients that can be served in the four-hour time block, as is seen in Figure 9.1. It shows that flights of four patients get most of the way there, about 18 patients.

But what happens to patient satisfaction as the flights get bigger? Well, it goes down. If flights of four patients are booked, then patient 4, after being prepped, can figure on waiting 30 minutes before actually seeing the doctor. Using a simple model that says patient satisfaction drops one point for every minute of waiting beyond 10 minutes, patient satisfaction would go as seen in Figure 9.2. This is a heuristic model offered for illustration.[2]

---

2. There are studies in the literature of how long patients will wait before getting mad enough to walk away. There are few, if any, studies of increasing anger short of walking away. Lacking an evidence-based model, we offer a heuristic model in order to illustrate the general point. *Heuristic* means we made it up out of whole cloth.

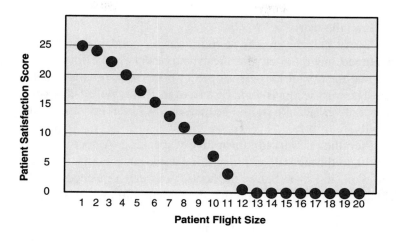

Figure 9.2   Patient satisfaction versus flight size.

Wow! Pretty clear trade-off, with patient satisfaction dropping like a rock. Looks like the right answer is to book flights of three patients to get some productivity without driving patients away, and maybe experiment with flights of four to see how patients react. Maybe think of something else for the fourth patients to be doing, such as being interviewed by a doctor's assistant or contributing to a patient survey. (Maybe not a survey on waiting times, though.)

REDUCE VARIABILITY

The variability in the treatment time contributes to lost productivity. Reducing variability allows closer booking and increases capacity and revenue.

The scheduling rule being used here is based on the mean treatment time plus twice the standard deviation of the treatment time. Reducing the standard deviation by a minute is worth twice as much as reducing the mean by a minute.

Therefore, focus on reducing the *variability* in the treatment time.

There are two kinds of variability here, as there always are, controllable variability and uncontrollable variability. Go to work on the controllable variability.

Prep the work.

Verify that the treatment room has all conceivable supplies in plentitude, that the doctor has fresh batteries in every electronic gizmo, and that the doctor has a fresh prescription pad and a new ballpoint pen. This verification should be an assigned duty with a checklist, and the act of verification should be tracked just like every other managed activity.

Prep the patient, administratively speaking. A doctor's assistant should go through all administrative items such as insurance, transportation, and so on before the doctor goes in. Use a checklist. Track. This reduces the likelihood that the patient will ask questions about these things of the doctor, which takes up doctor-time.

Manage interruptions. Telephone calls to the doctor are important; however, not every telephone call needs to be taken in real time. Messaging works. Carrying calls over to the next buffer time slot works, provided that the carryover time does not seem unreasonable to the caller.

Nonpatient calls should be handled by messaging. The point of customer service is to serve customers, and time given to nonpatients merits a lower urgency.

Patient calls should be treated with kindly attention, even if they are going to result in a callback or a relaying of messages. This needs a script. Get a phone number immediately just in case the call is lost. Cross-check phone numbers against those on file as a check against error in stating or recording the number. Take control of the sequence of encounters. Do positive follow-up, even if there is nothing helpful to report.

For those patients who call and have messages relayed to them from the doctor, it is a positive thing for the doctor to call the patient personally later on, when time permits, to reconfirm the message and regenerate personal contact. The whole point is to provide customer service in order to build patient loyalty.

LATE-SHOWS

The flight-of-three or flight-of-four scheduling plan has a built-in tolerance for patients who show up a little late.

However, it is a principle of Six Sigma that the target must always be the nominal value, not the just-barely value. See Chapter 19, page 125 for Six Sigma design rules.

The reason for this is simple. If just-barely is tolerated at all, the whole system degenerates to just-barely, which makes for raggedy performance. So, late-shows need to be remediated in every instance.

Every late-show should get a standard interview. Was the time known? Was it transportation? Was it a third party? Was it forgetfulness? Was it illness? And so on. What will be different next time? How is this going to be prevented from happening again?

Lateness causes should be charted and tracked, looking for patterns and clusters. There may even be common causes, such as erratic van service from particular long-term care facilities. Perhaps these can be remedied.

Now, if the lateness doesn't preclude joining the assigned flight, there is a strategic question of whether to take the patient in or rebook the patient for a later date. This is ultimately a game of chicken, so there should be a firm policy. The policy should probably be that any patient will be sent home on the second and any subsequent late-show.

There also needs to be a definition of *on time*. Is there a grace period of one minute? Five minutes? The only coherent policy is no, there is no grace period. Be in queue to register by the appointed minute or go into the lateness remediation drill.

EARLY-SHOWS

Patients who show up quite early are only a problem to the extent that increasing the body count in the waiting room gives others the impression that the office doesn't run on schedule. Putting early-shows on one side of the waiting room under a big sign saying "early arrivers" probably doesn't work toward an overall benefit.

The stern policy is to make early arrivers wait to encourage them to believe the schedule the next time. That may not work and does not address the waiting room crowding issue.

The practical policy is to fit them into the schedule ahead of time if an opening presents itself. This helps clear the waiting room, even at the risk of encouraging the patient to come even earlier the next time. Maybe give the person a token reward for accepting the early action time. That goes in the direction of encouraging early-shows, so the reward needs to be kept to the token level.

This is self-queuing. Queuing is more efficient than nonqueuing, and, in this case, it is the patient who is volunteering to wait in queue.

One important thing, though, is to make sure the patient knows that it is the patient who is creating the queue, that the patient knew the original booking time, and that the patient's next booking is completely understood and documented.

NO-SHOWS

No-shows are the bane of scheduled service.

The no-show is a loss of revenue, even if the no-show is rebooked for a later date. There is a time-value to revenue, and revenue postponed is worth less than revenue earned this day.

Moreover, there is an opportunity cost (risk of exclusion of future revenue) for every rebooked patient, because that future booking slot is then no longer available for the booking of an additional patient. Rebooking no-shows causes a disadvantageous ripple effect.

Make reminder calls in advance to reduce the likelihood of no-shows.

In addition, anticipate that no-shows are apt to be an issue (which can be quantified based on prior experience), and plan accordingly by identifying patients ahead of time who have flexibility and who can be pulled forward on short notice. Give such patients a token reward of some kind if they are called in early.

Make a target of having two possible pull-ins identified for every statistically-likely no-show, day for day. Or to be more elegant about it, identify enough flexible patients so that there is a 95 percent likelihood that all slots will be occupied. (List the number of no-shows for like periods, such as Friday mornings. Calculate the mean value for that list. Calculate the standard deviation for that list.[3] Add

---

3. *Average* and *standard deviation* are built-in spreadsheet functions. See Appendix A, page 205, which includes common spreadsheet functions.

twice the standard deviation to the mean, giving an estimate of the number of no-shows that will not be exceeded more than five percent of the time.)

Pulling patients *forward* in time is positive. It helps the present value of revenue by bringing that revenue forward. It creates an opportunity to book some other patient into the future slot just vacated. It's positive.

10

Bottlenecks

A bottleneck is the part of the system that has limited capacity compared to demand; that cannot easily or economically be expanded; and that limits overall production in an important way. In multistep processes, effective production planning means getting upstream planning right so the bottleneck stays busy.

CHECKLIST

☑ The production of the bottleneck is the production of the system.

☑ Plan from the bottleneck in both directions.

☑ Restrain bottleneck commitment to allow for catch-up.

☑ Work to improve the bottleneck capacity.

☑ If there are steps upstream of the bottleneck, focus attention on upstream operations.

BACKGROUND

The bottleneck may be an expensive machine, such as an MRI machine or a PET scanner. The bottleneck may be the physical size of a room or building. The bottleneck may be the number of surgical nurses available. The bottleneck may be the number of beds allowed by a regulatory agency. The bottleneck may be an administrative limit.

Virtually every organization has a bottleneck.[1] Managing production through the bottleneck is key to managing production for the entire organization.

FIRST-POSITION BOTTLENECK

Let's look at the simplest situation, a bottleneck at the first step in a process. For example, consider a freestanding service that does MRI scans, organizes the data, and ships the data to the primary care physician. The capacity limit is the MRI machine itself, which is in the first position on the flowchart in Figure 10.1.

Since it is given that the first step is the bottleneck, it follows that the subsequent steps are not bottlenecks. It is virtually impossible to have two bottlenecks in one system. If the bottleneck is in the first position, then all the downstream steps are not bottlenecks. Since they are not bottlenecks, they have more production capacity than the bottleneck does (or else one of them would be the bottleneck). Since they have more capacity, if something happens to interfere with their production for a limited time, they can catch up again. Overall production is not inhibited.

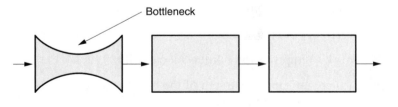

Figure 10.1   Flowchart with bottleneck in first position.

---

1. An organization that does not have a bottleneck is deploying excess capacity and should take steps to reduce capacity, stimulate demand, or both.

The upshot is that, with the bottleneck in the first position, planning for this multistep process boils down to planning for the first step alone. The others can fend for themselves.

What's more, the downstream steps will be idle part of the time, starved for work. That is necessarily true, since they have more capacity than the bottleneck does. That's okay, they *should* be idle part of the time, given these circumstances.

All of the previous discussion of matching populations and capacity, queuing and nonqueuing, scheduled, mixed, and nonscheduled work still applies, considering the bottleneck by itself.

The Honda Rule

It is said that Honda has a rule. Honda does not commit more than 80 percent of the production of any of its car factories. That way, if something happens to interfere with production, the factory has surge capacity to catch up.

Consider the alternative. Losses of production cannot be avoided 100 percent of the time, year after year, so if the factory were committed to 100 percent of its nominal capacity, it follows that the factory would fall behind plan every time there is an outage and never catch up. Honda figures that being unable to plan its business downstream of the factory is a bigger burden than having 20 percent of the factory standing idle most of the time (or all of the factory standing idle 20 percent of the time).

That's an interesting business decision. At face value, it entails a lower return on productive assets than would otherwise apply. On the other hand, if Honda's experience is that various things come along and shut down production about 10 percent of the time, than the give-up is perhaps 10 percent of return on those assets rather than the nominal 20 percent give-up. Honda is paying something, in terms of lower return, in order to get a higher certainty in product flow throughout its system.

Planning-in some reserve bottleneck capacity is good business strategy.

Should it be 20 percent? A systematic approach would be to track downtime and figure out a capacity reserve that covers unplanned outages to at least 95 percent confidence.

Note that the capacity reserve applies only to the bottleneck unit. All other units already have slack and don't need any more.

IMPROVING BOTTLENECK PRODUCTION

The bottleneck will go idle if there is no work to be done. Precluding this unhappy state of affairs means having patients all prepped, qualified, and ready to go. All the previous discussion of patient scheduling, having on-call standby patients, and coping with no-shows, applies.

The work done in the bottleneck can be improved by working on the mean execution time and the controllable variability of the time required in the bottleneck. This includes team training, supplies management, setup, room arrangement, and all other things that contribute to upsets or nonideal operations.

FALSE BOTTLENECKS

In real life, it happens that bottlenecks are discovered where no one expects them to be. An MRI service may be jammed up for lack of a sufficient number of dressing rooms. So, build more dressing rooms.

After all the trivial matters are cleared away, the real, immovable bottleneck will stand in stark relief. See Figure 10.2.

SECOND-POSITION BOTTLENECK

Now let's consider a system where the bottleneck is not in the first position, but rather in the second position. See Figure 10.3. For example, consider the case where orthopedic surgery is followed by skilled nursing care, and the bottleneck is a chronic scarcity of skilled nursing beds. Let's presume that the surgery is not urgent so that patient scheduling can be done freely. If there are third, fourth, and other steps downstream of the bottleneck, then they will have

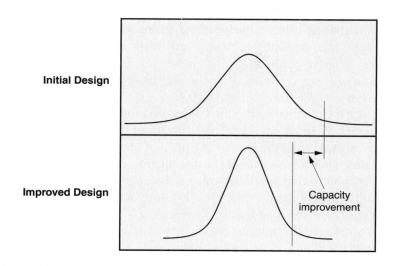

Figure 10.2 Capacity increase due to reduced variability.

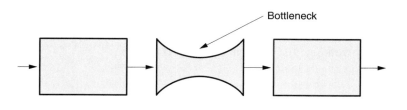

Figure 10.3 Flowchart with bottleneck in second position.

capacity to catch up if they are stalled for some reason, so they don't need any attention here. If they get behind, they can catch up. They will be idle part of the time, on purpose.

The issue at hand is, how does one deal with the upstream steps in production?

What is known at this point is that, by comparison to the capacity of the bottleneck, the capacity of the upstream step is large. The upstream step will be idle part of the time.

It is also known that the upstream step can lose production because of some upset in its own operation or for lack of work to do (no patient on hand, most likely). If the upstream step fails to produce its output, then the bottleneck will run out of work, and the whole system will lose production. That's bad. Yet, it cannot be excluded that this will happen to the upstream step once in a while.

What to do? Consider Figure 10.4.

Since the point is to keep the bottleneck producing, the first thing is to define an *inventory level* just upstream of the bottleneck. That's an inventory of patients. How many patients should be in inventory? Enough so that it is very unlikely that this inventory level will go to zero, because at that point the bottleneck would run out of work.

To figure out the inventory level, figure out how many patients are 'consumed' per hour by the bottleneck, and figure out how long the longest credible nonproduction time is for the upstream step. "Longest credible" might correspond to, say, 95 percent of previous outage experience. Then, multiply that longest credible upstream nonproduction time by the bottleneck's consumption rate and that gives the inventory level, expressed in patient count.

To work a simple case: suppose the bottleneck consumes four patients per hour and the 95 percent confidence level upstream outage is 0.75 hours. Multiply to get three, the number of patients to be held in inventory just upstream of the bottleneck.

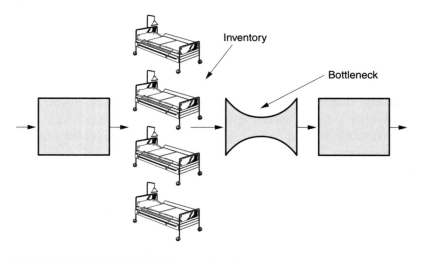

Figure 10.4 Flowchart with inventory before bottleneck.

There are several implications of this that may be worth considering.

The upstream step runs 45 minutes in advance of the bottleneck in normal production. That is to say, there will three patients in inventory at all normal times. If the inventory goes up to four, the upstream step should shut down, at least briefly. If the inventory goes down to two, then the upstream step should hurry up, use some of its excess capacity, and get the inventory level back up to three.

So, the upstream step runs in start-stop mode, and its starting and stopping are not governed by the bottleneck but rather by the inventory level. Upstream and bottleneck are decoupled by the existence of the inventory.

This mode of operation for the upstream step has its own name. It's called *kanban*, and it can be shown to be the optimum production method for any combination of production steps upstream of a bottleneck. The word kanban is an anglicized version of a Japanese word for a punched card, because the inventory boss would instruct the upstream production boss to start production again, inventory being low, by passing a punched card. Or so the story goes.

Since we are talking about inventory while meaning patients in the process of being treated, and considering that sitting or lying there for 45 minutes in our case is unlikely to be an attractive feature of the service, it is worth a moment to consider how to reduce the inventory. If the inventory could be reduced by half, the queuing time (the time in inventory) would be reduced by 22.5 minutes, and the total treatment cycle experienced by every patient would be reduced by 22.5 minutes.

The inventory time is determined entirely by the upstream step's recovery time. How long does it take the upstream step to recover from any and all upsets? What physical improvements would reduce recovery time? Could spare equipment be built in with quick or automatic fail-over? Could incentives be given to patients so that fill-in patients are at hand in case of a no-show? Could testing be built in to the upstream step so that any patient needing a second pass through the upstream step could be restarted immediately?

Note that there is no direct incentive to reduce the mean or variance in the production time for the upstream step, which has spare capacity by definition. All (well, let's say, most) attention should be applied in the upstream step to improving upstream recovery time.

YIELD

Factories figure on some product being lost in each step of production, so they start with extra feedstock. That thinking doesn't work in healthcare, since the 'feedstock' is a patient. Any patient starting through the treatment expects to go all the way through.

Even so, it is possible that a patient will be found to be unsuited for further treatment when the patient is at the beginning or partway through. If the patient is at the beginning, this is the same, for production purposes, as a no-show. How to cope with no-shows was discussed earlier.

If the patient has passed through the bottleneck and is then found to be unsuitable for further treatment, then one unit of production has been misspent and cannot be recovered. Too bad.

If the patient has begun treatment and is still upstream of the bottleneck, then the effect of dropping this patient out of the treatment process is the same as an outage of the upstream step. The upstream step needs to recover. This is the same as an upstream machine outage of comparable time. The upstream stage has excess capacity, compared to the bottleneck, so the upstream stage will catch up.

Any dropout of a patient anywhere in the treatment process has a negative impact, so there is merit in paying attention to qualifying the patient for treatment entirely beforehand, before any productive effort at all has been applied to that patient. That is not only good production management, it's compassionate common sense.

Moreover, if a patient is to be dropped from the treatment process, the place to do it is upstream of the bottleneck, because the upstream step has the possibility of recovery, and the inventory just ahead of the bottleneck provides a bit of a buffer.

PERSPECTIVE ON QUEUING AND BOTTLENECKS

There is quite a nice study available online (KPMG 2002) on patient dissatisfaction with queuing times in the United Kingdom. The questions posed in the survey of patients had to do with patient satisfaction given that the patients were waiting *three months* or *six months* for treatment after doctor's referral. Nice glossy presentation by the consultant, replete with pie charts, but not the kind of service Americans are going to want.

Operations

11
Global Optimization

The service line manager identifies with a population of patients served in order to have the global perspective. The service line manager has to have financial responsibility or else no one will pay any attention to him or her.

CHECKLIST

- ☑ Optimize globally in favor of patients.
- ☑ Service line manager identifies with a population of patients.
- ☑ Service line manager has profit and loss responsibility.
- ☑ Others, such as department heads, do not have profit responsibility.

OBJECTIVES OF THE ORGANIZATION

The patients' objectives were stated earlier, page 7, as these:

- Outcomes consistent with national standards

- Attentive care

- Consideration of the patient's time

The organization's objectives need to be consistent with the patient's objectives or else the patient will find a more responsive care provider.

A consistent set of objectives for the organization are:

1. Treatment for all patients consistent with national standards

2. Attentive care for all patients

3. Effective use of resources

4. Sustainable financials

The first two of these follow directly from the patient's objectives. The latter two objectives for the organization are self-evident. Not trivial by any means, but self-evident. The organization can only serve the patient population over the long run if it survives over the short run.

IDENTIFYING WITH PATIENTS

Since the organization's objectives follow from the patient's objectives, it follows that the organization needs to assign management responsibility to connect the organization to patient populations.

One popular means for doing this is to create service line managers (Gee 2003).

We endorse service line managers, and we make two additional recommendations:

1. The service line manager is assigned a patient *population.*

2. The service line manager is assigned profit and loss responsibility.

The first of these, identifying with a population, is important for any service industry. The service line manager must be in touch with, must talk to, must listen to, must identify with a population of patients (customers) to understand the purpose and benefit of the service offered as viewed by that population. The focus must be external. There are plenty of other people looking out for internal matters, so somebody—namely the service line manager—needs to be thinking about the externals and seeing things from the perspective of the patient.

There is no point in looking out for the patient population, though, unless the service line has sustainable financials, and therefore the service line must be a profit center.[1]

Therefore, both of these responsibilities need to be assigned to the same person, the service line manager. Assigning them to different people would only add the need for a third person to resolve the tensions between them.

The population focus does not start with admission and end with discharge. Rather, the population focus abides. Many patients have chronic conditions and are apt to be readmitted later on. Given the payment schemes used these days, a patient readmitted too soon may not bring new revenue. The service line manager may find it important to understand how home health and other postdischarge services are being provided and how patients are connecting with support groups after discharge.

For elderly populations, many admissions come from long-term care facilities. If the long-term care facility is not providing high standards of care, there may be not only an impact on the well-being of the patient, there can be a negative impact on the hospital. For example, if the long-term care facility is not being careful in assuring sufficient patient movement to preclude pressure ulcers, the patient may be admitted to the hospital for other reasons, with an incipient pressure ulcer condition. If the pressure ulcer then manifests itself during the hospital stay, the hospital can probably not discharge the patient back to the long-term care facility until the pressure ulcer is cleared up. Nor is the hospital likely to find much revenue to pay for this added treatment.

An extension of this postdischarge interest is the current national interest in 'disease management' (CMS 2004) for chronic conditions

---

1. Substitute *contribution margin center* or other euphemism to match the local usage.

such as diabetes, heart conditions, and the like. The idea is that patients who take care of themselves require less acute care. Disease management programs have care-advisors in touch with the target population to urge better self-care. This may work. On the other hand, it is not yet obvious that nagging people with chronic conditions makes them take care of themselves any better than leaving them alone, given that they already know what they are supposed to be doing for themselves. As regards service line management, if disease management has little impact on the population, then the service line of business is unchanged. On the other hand, if disease management turns out to be successful for some populations, the informed service line manager is positioned to adapt the service line to the new market conditions. Indeed, in that case, the service line manager may strive to find a new stream of revenue for providing the disease management service, which some insurance payers are now supporting on a trial basis (Landro 2003).

The service line manager doing outreach can address operational issues such as patient identification by such means as coordinating wristband identification systems with long-term care facilities or establishing biometric identification systems compatible with long-term care facilities and community programs.

FINANCIAL RESPONSIBILITY

Consider the profit center responsibility. Since most hospitals have more than one service line, there will be a competition for resources and capital money between the profit centers. That's healthy and normal; it occurs in all business organizations.

Consider the service line manager for outpatient surgery. Surgeons decide sometimes to keep a patient for observation. At this writing, Medicare and other payers pay so poorly for 'observation' that most acute care hospitals lose money on observation cases. A service line manager upon learning this can consider various courses of action on a financial reward basis. Accept the loss, hoping to make it up in future business; refuse to admit the patient; tell the physician to write a standard admissions order or take the patient elsewhere.

Some community hospitals now take the third of these, finding that the physician just rewrites the admission order to make it a standard admission. This takes care of the patient, and it solves a financial problem.

Having a service line manager analyzing the financial aspects is a means to identify such cost/payment clashes to bring them to senior management for policy review.

If the service line manager is not given *profit* responsibility, then the natural tendency is for the service line manager to argue for more services for the particular population without consideration of cost. That's not workable in the long run because resources would get allocated to the cleverest talker rather than the best performer. Other measures of performance, such as market share, tend to go in this same unfavorable direction.

SUPPORT DEPARTMENTS

If the service lines are profit centers, other departments such as X-ray, laboratory, and pharmacy *cannot* be profit centers. If the pharmacy, for instance, were a profit center, then the pharmacy would be driven to optimizing its service for itself. That's bad. The need is to optimize globally, which is to say optimize for the patient. The pharmacy is not apt to have that global perspective inherently, nor would any of the other support departments.

Such departments need to be evaluated and incentivized on measures of service rendered to the service lines, thence to the patients, and on their efficiency in rendering the service, but efficiency has to rank below effectiveness.

Naturally, such departments can provide even higher levels of service if they have more money to spend. Given that the total amount of money available is finite, there needs to be a trade-off between level of service and cost. The point here is that this trade-off must be made on a global, patient-perspective basis, not on a department by department basis. That global perspective abides in the service line managers. Competition for resources should be between product line managers, each of whom can marshal facts and population-based projections.

SERVICE LINE MANAGER SELECTION

It is to be noted that service line managers have a business role, not a medical role, to play. The right background for a service line manager is in hospital administration or in service sales in the general field of healthcare. A background in case management might be the very thing, coupled with the appropriate personal skills and career interests.

12

Utilization

Getting high utilization rates requires continual attention by expediters charged with clearing away encumbrances that arise spontaneously in any organization.

CHECKLIST

☑ Track value added.

☑ Eliminate local optima.

☑ Expedite.

RESOURCES AND UTILIZATION

In acute care, patients are commonly provided with laboratory analysis, X-ray, medications, bed rest, and other services. The patient stays until a discharge order is written. Several different departments and persons need to act in a timely manner if the patient is to be discharged as soon as the medically necessary time is elapsed.

In Figure 12.1, the long slanted line shows that a certain amount of time is considered to be medically necessary for the particular diagnosis. Precision is not required, just an estimate, for present purposes.

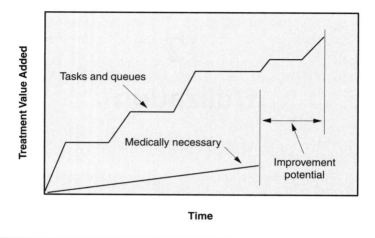

Figure 12.1 Optimizing treatment time.

The segmented line shows value being added when the line segments go up, and no value being added when the line is flat. This could be time spent waiting for the X-ray department to do an X-ray for this patient, or it could be time spent waiting for the doctor to write the discharge order. Every one of those flat line segments is a candidate for improvement.

While there is no point in reducing the flat line segments beyond the point where the medically-necessary line becomes limiting, there is every incentive to get to that point and maybe a little further, just to be on the good side.

It is in the interest of the patient to get the treatment completed as soon as possible, so global optimization in favor of the patient is reached when the medically-necessary line is limiting.

LOCAL OPTIMIZATION

The flat line segments in Figure 12.1 indicate that local optimization is happening. For instance, consider time waiting for lab results to be returned. One of the flat lines might represent time waiting for a lab technician to finish prior work before taking up this patient's lab work. That flat line could be shortened by adding lab technicians to increase the lab capacity. The present number of lab technicians may represent the least-average-cost technician count, meaning that all the lab techs are almost always busy (a bottleneck caused by a staffing rule). Is that the right overall policy? Perhaps. Or perhaps adding lab techs or techs on weekend shifts or something else would provide better facility utilization even though the cost of operating the laboratory would be higher because lab techs would be idle from time to time or being paid at a premium rate.

Consider the time spent waiting for the attending physician to sign the discharge order. Some hospitals issue laptop computers with wireless Internet access or personal digital assistants to reduce this wait time.

Consider the time spent finding a skilled nursing home to take the patient. Could this special need have been known and dealt with before the patient was admitted?

What to Do

Make value-added charts. Look for flat lines and patterns.

Given that acute care stays are now so short, and getting shorter, it is vital that the discharge plan for each patient be established before the patient is admitted. For instance, to the extent that the need for a skilled nursing bed cannot be determined before admission, but one may be needed, then contingency plans should be made so that one will be available if needed.

That won't work for unscheduled admissions of previously-unknown patients, but even for this population the discharge planning team can be triggered at the moment of admission to minimize the risk of delay in discharging.

Expedite. Assign expediters, preferably case managers, charged with the responsibility of knowing the status of care for each patient, knowing what support service work, such as lab and X-ray, is awaited, and staying in touch with all departments to find any holdups. Even the best organizations with the best of intentions need expediters.

CASE MANAGER AS EXPEDITER

Case management, in the purest sense, is concerned with the case-by-case delivery of patient care by providers; case management commonly is combined with processes such as utilization review/ management, discharge planning, orchestration of individualized care for select patient cases, and cost containment (Wojner 2001, 11).

While that is a fine purpose, some hospitals have made additional use of the case manager, who is typically a registered nurse, to expedite the provision of care.

Expediting is keeping everything moving, making phone calls, finding the doctor to sign the discharge order, and so on, for each patient.

Case managers, working with service line managers, can develop improvements to the standard care plans to allow improvement that will show up on the value-added charts. For instance, preadmission interviews and patient/family training sessions may identify discharge needs before admission or special handling requirements if, say, the patient is coming in for a knee operation but has one arm in a sling because of an unrelated injury. Better to know such things beforehand.

MEDICAL RECORD COMPLETENESS

The other part of the expediting is to expedite completeness of the medical record so that the case can be coded and sent to the payer for payment.

This includes expediting the attending physician to get any dictation done, checking to see that the record includes all the billable services, and checking to see that the medical record is stated in the proper way for collection.

For instance, a record saying *septicemia* may justify higher payment than a record saying *urosepsis*, even if the two words are describing the same physical condition. The physician may not be sensitive to this point, since hospital reimbursement does not touch the physician directly. Somebody has to look out for the hospital's interest in such things. Therefore, it is a reasonable role for the case manager to scan for such hot-button words and ask the physician if the preferred word can be used instead.

This optimizes in the hospital's direction at no cost to the patient and addresses the hospital's objective of financial stability. The patient is not held beyond the medically necessary time, and the institution is paid according to the established rules.

THE MEDICALLY NECESSARY TREATMENT TIME

It is up to the medical staff to determine the medically necessary treatment time. Since this sets the minimum time the patient will be in treatment, this is the objective time-point for improving the process, getting rid of the slack, and tightening up the process.

Once the improvement is accomplished, it is natural to ask the doctor or doctors if the medically necessary treatment time can be reduced. This is an occasion to apply Toyota Rule 14 (Liker 2004). Toyota Rule 14 is to ask *why?* five times.

Why? Why? Why? Why? Why?

This is quite annoying after about the third why, so some stealth is in order. Ask the way a Japanese would, applying infinite politeness.

"Can you help me understand this, please?"

"That's very interesting. Can you explain this point a little more, please?"

"Hmm. And then what does this mean?"

And so on.

The logic underlying this repetition is that the first couple of answers will be rote, responsive, but not revealing. Asking five times drives the askee to the point of reflecting deeply on the point. Why exactly is it that this is so?

The hope is that the askee, upon reflection, will come up with ways of reducing the medically necessary time while preserving all aspects of patient safety and care.

Unasked, the askee may have little incentive to think of ways to reduce the time. What's more, asking politely is more apt to bear fruit than twisting arms.

This is Rule 14 of the Toyota management rules. The others are interesting, too, and are given in the same reference.

13

Magnet Nursing

*Attract nurses by adopting the management practices known
to attract nurses like a magnet.*

CHECKLIST

☑ The chief nursing officer is a member of the senior
management council.

☑ Nursing management is consulted on operational matters.

☑ Nurses are treated like the professionals they are.

THE MAGNET CONCEPT

With nurses being in impossibly short supply, employers are faced
with entering an auction to hire nurses to make good on turnover or
finding ways to reduce turnover.

To reduce turnover, make yours a place that attracts, and does
not repel, nurses.

There is a guidebook for this (ANA 2003).

There are some key points for management to consider. To begin, the chief nursing officer (CNO) should be in the same senior management councils as the chief medical officer, the chief financial officer, and so on—equal ranking on the organization chart. Moreover, the interests of the senior nursing manager should not be diluted by having this person responsible for ancillary departments such as pharmacy or X-ray; nursing deserves its own seat at the senior management council table.

Since the nursing staff operates the patient care part of the institution, nursing management should participate in all management deliberations related thereto.

The nursing staffing model should be consistent with the professional and legal responsibilities of the nurses.

Expectations for nursing performance should be consistent with resources provided. In particular, long shifts are a bad idea. Responsibility for too many patients is a bad idea.[1]

NURSING STAFFING MODELS

There are three models in common use in acute care hospitals these days: the all-RN model, the RN-team model, and the care-pair model.

We do not recommend the RN-team model for reasons which will be explained. We do recommend the all-RN model and the care-pair model.

The All-RN Model

The all-RN model is frequently used in critical care units and in other specialized units where it is expected that many professional decisions and actions will be required per patient and per hour.

The all-RN model is also used in some teaching and university hospitals in medical/surgical units, partly because there is an abundance of RNs.

---

1. At this writing, both of these are subjects for legislation in some states to rectify what the public perceives to be bad practices.

The all-RN model has much to recommend it. Every person, since each is an RN, is qualified to deal with every eventuality. All patient contacts are with someone, an RN, who can respond with professional competence. This goes in the direction of improved patient perception of service, as discussed earlier in Chapter 6.

A version of this is the "rich BSN" model, in which many RNs are qualified to the bachelors level rather than merely to the diploma level. While both kinds of nurses are licensed in the same way, the BSN nurse has a higher level of education in the course of disease and patient response and can be expected to understand patient progress in a deeper context. The rich BSN model correlates with better patient outcomes. See (Weinberg 2003, 13) for elaboration of this point with additional references.

The RN-Team Model

The team model became popular about 50 years ago. The team consists of one RN and several nurse assistants with lower qualifications. The underlying idea is that the RN supervises the others, and the others act to multiply the reach of the RN.

While this might have been an effective model in those bygone days when lots of people in an acute care hospital were there for recuperation and weren't all that sick, it doesn't work today. The specific deficiencies are these:

1. The nurse has little or no authority over the team members and cannot in practice tell them what to do or when to do it.

2. The nurse is legally and professionally responsible for work that is done out of sight and not entirely under the nurse's control. This is unprofessional at best.

3. The law of stratified labor grades (see page 57) says that the RN alone has to deal with nearly all unpredictable events, which are all the more numerous now since all patients are actually sick.

4. The same law of stratified labor grades says that the support team members will be idle intermittently even while the RN is overworked, vitiating any labor cost savings that might have been. (Weinberg 2003, 67).

For these reasons, we believe that the RN-team model is no longer functional and is not appropriate for Magnet Nursing.

The Care-Pair Model

The care-pair model, as has been practiced by Cleveland Clinic, assigns one assistant to each RN, and the pair do all caregiving for their assigned patients together.

Because each patient interaction includes the nurse, the patient has frequent opportunity to get a qualified professional response and action if appropriate. This goes in the direction of improving the patient's perception of both service and care.

The nurse is in charge and responsible for the actions of the assistant, who stays within sight.

This model keeps the nurse in close contact with the patients, for whom the nurse is legally and professionally responsible. This model eliminates the chance that a nurse assistant, out of sight, will do something that is not consistent with the current state of the patient's treatment. This model gets productivity from the nurse assistant.

The assistant so assigned needs to be instructed by management to take orders from the nurse. The assistant is not a free agent and cannot have independent duties.

If the assistant is a student nurse, then working in this model with an experienced nurse gives the student an excellent opportunity to be tutored in real-life situations.

The care-pair model provides the patient with a nurse at every interaction and saves salary cost compared to the all-RN model.

We recommend the care-pair model.

14

Training and Retraining

Training and retraining are essential to the attainment of high and consistent performance. Everybody needs training. Everybody needs retraining.

CHECKLIST

☑ Train a few people in specific Six Sigma skills.

☑ Make management aware of Six Sigma concepts.

☑ Train your own people rather than relying on consultants.

SIX SIGMA TRAINING *PER SE*

Not everyone needs to be an expert in Six Sigma. Most managers and professionals need awareness; operations managers need specific instruction. A small number, perhaps one percent of the professional staff, need 20 to 50 hours of skills training together with project implementation experience.[1] At least one senior manager

---

1. Success is rewarded by recognition as Six Sigma Green Belt and Black Belt proficiency. See page 3.

should be trained to this level. (Some corporations, notably GE, now require management candidates, even for the mailroom, to have some level of qualification in Six Sigma.)

The Six Sigma training can be done by a contractor or by a member of the in-house training staff. Most outside training companies think in factory terms and are not much help; however, there are some training firms that have specialized in healthcare and can provide apt training programs. Usually, outside contractor training is used only as a bridge, with in-house training taking over as soon as the in-house training staff gets a solid footing. Tables 14.1, 14.2, and 14.3 give topics to be understood at each level.

Table 14.1 Awareness level—most professionals.

Topics	Reference page
Flowcharts	177
Design of tasks against inadvertent error	147
Gates, buffers, system design basics	123, 151,155
Variability, controllable and uncontrollable	8
Tracking charts	163
Bathtub curve	102

Table 14.2 Operational level—most line managers.

Topics	Reference page
Defense in depth	129
Three-plane causal analysis	185
Blame-free workplace	102
Visualization techniques	26
Sequential event analysis	235
Capacity analysis	35, 73

Table 14.3 Senior level—most senior managers.

Topics	Reference page
Global optimization in favor of patients	83
Evidence-based medicine policy	11
Service line management	197
Magnet nursing	95
Variability, controllable and uncontrollable	8
Bathtub curve	102
Blame-free workplace	102
Capacity analysis	35, 73

RETRAINING

Disaster Drills

Annual disaster drills are commonly practiced on the basis of a hurricane or tornado, carrying things as far as moving patients away from windows and the like. These are fine, but they are not very frequent, and since they are a group activity, their value wanes as the group changes over the months.

Supplement annual drills with quarterly walk-throughs to refresh memories and to bring new group members into the fold.

Just-in-Time Updates

The best time to do retraining is at the very moment of application. This can be as simple as an activity leader reminding the group of what's to be done next. Or, for example, a nurse who is about to do a titration, not having done one for two years, rereads the manual or rewatches the vendor's videotape.

Any care provider of any rank should be encouraged to ask to be refreshed on how to do an unfamiliar task. Better to refresh than . . . .

Corrective Retraining

If an error is made, the appropriate corrective action in a blame-free workplace is to retrain the person who made the error. This does two things. First of all, it conveys the message that errors are not to be taken lightly. Second, it conveys the message that the person is not being blamed but rather encouraged to improve. It's not the person at fault, it's the system, particularly the training component of the system that got stale for this particular person. That's not as circular as it sounds because the person did not set out to make the error, but made the error nonetheless.

People follow the *bathtub curve*. People make mistakes when learning a new skill, naturally. Then follows a sustained period when the rate of mistake making is very low. Later, bad habits or forgetfulness creep in. The important thing is that this is perfectly natural and happens to everybody. Airline pilots do periodic retraining in flight simulators, under the watchful eye of an instructor, even though they fly the same model of plane every day. The simulator exercises include practice for emergencies, but they also include the routine tasks of getting the airplane off the ground and back down again.

Note the bathtub curve illustration in Figure 14.1. The error rate is high at both ends, low in the middle. Initial training works on the left end of the curve, getting the error rate down in the first place. Periodic retraining applies in the middle and anticipates that bad habits or forgetfulness lurk. Corrective retraining works on the right end of the curve, getting people back to the middle.

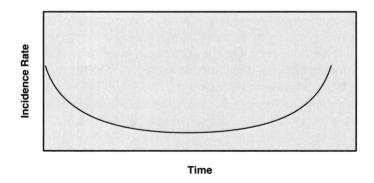

Figure 14.1 Bathtub curve.

15

Autoremediation

Posting tracking charts does wonders for self-improvement. This applies to physicians, technicians, laborers, individuals, and groups. And it's free!

CHECKLIST

☑ Define significant performance parameters.

☑ Track and post.

☑ Let nature take its course.

SELF-ESTEEM AS MOTIVATOR

In any modern organization, people manage themselves. The senior management issue is to get people to manage themselves in the right direction to support optimization in favor of patients. That requires communications in the downward direction. It's also helpful if management has some way of knowing what's going on, how well things are going, and where the issues are. More communications needed, this time in the upward direction.

Six Sigma encourages the use of tracking charts as the communications tool.

Tracking charts track items that management thinks are important. While this may seem to be trite, the fact is that organizational studies almost always find that employees have only the vaguest idea of what management thinks to be important.

Tracking charts show performance.

The performers see immediately how well things are going. The performers may be employees, they may be independent physicians, they may be contractors. They may be groups or subgroups, such as shift workers.

The natural response, after getting over the idea of being measured at all, is to try to do better, to get a higher score.

A community hospital chief medical officer remarked to the authors that tracking charts work particularly well with physicians because they are naturally competitive. If scores are being kept, every physician wants the top score. Considering that most community hospital physicians are not employees of the hospital and that the hospital has very little leverage over nonemployee physicians, getting the physicians to be self-motivated is great.

It all goes to optimizing, globally, in favor of the patient.

Figure 15.1 shows a simple tracking chart, with no direct identification of the participants, only code names. This is enough, provided that each of the participants knows his or her own code name.

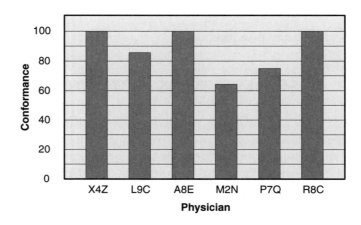

Figure 15.1 Use of preferred protocol.

The idea is to get self-motivation going, and for that, the participant need only know that score is being kept and that a high score is better than a low score.

The simple tracking chart example in Figure 15.1 could be embellished a bit by adding a line at the level corresponding to the objective. However, the self-motivation phenomenon works whether there is an objective line or not. The self-motivation is simply to make the particular ribbon go up. All the way up.

When applied to teams, the psychology is the same. Even if the members of the team are not particularly in sync with one another, there is a powerful tendency to put aside individuality and focus on team improvement.

Tracking charts are the starting point for almost all Six Sigma improvement projects because they contribute to an understanding of what's actually going on.

LOWER-STANDING TOPICS

Tracking charts and self-motivation are of interest to senior management when applied to key strategic issues.

Tracking charts and self-motivation are of interest to middle management when applied to operational issues.

Tracking charts and self-motivation are of interest to supervisory management for both of these reasons plus one more. Tracking charts are a painless way to get people to take care of those ordinary duties that tend to fall victim to higher-priority matters. Nagging doesn't work because the worker has a valid response, being busy with higher-priority work.

Consider, as an example, a nuclear medicine group that receives isotope shipments at various times, including during the off shifts. The group does an excellent job of receiving the special materials, keeping vaults locked, and getting the right isotope to the right patient. The group formerly had a clerk who kept the local inventory records, but the clerk went away in a prior cost-cutting campaign, so the technicians have been expected to record the deliveries in the local inventory log. Since they have had plenty of other things to do, all of which are more directly identified with patient care, those log entries were often forgotten. And yet, considering the special nature of the inventoried materials, the local log is not a frivolous matter. Non-logged deliveries were eventually discovered by working backwards from the physical inventory, but this was not timely nor necessarily complete.

Posting a tracking chart showing 'deliveries logged at delivery' over the vault worked better than a nagging sign, posted in the same place, saying "Post All Deliveries Immediately in the Inventory Record."

The problem went away, spontaneously, once the tracking chart was posted. (This was observed at a community hospital by one of the authors.)

16
Make or Buy

Medical transcription service provides an example of how to set standards and measure performance for support groups.

CHECKLIST

☑ Assert quantitative objectives.

☑ Set performance standards.

☑ Track and evaluate.

MAKE OR BUY SERVICES

Medical transcription services have traditionally been provided by hospitals to doctors. Doctors dictate, medical stenographers type, doctors correct, and the typescript goes into the patient's medical record.

For Medicare and many other insurance payers, the amount to be paid depends on what is in the patient's medical record, and the timing of payment depends on when the patient's medical record is completed and forwarded to the insurance coding department.

Both quality of the stenography and turnaround time count. Imperfect stenography means another lap around the dictate/type/ review circuit, which delays billing. That's bad.

Medical stenography has traditionally been handled as a staff service with only the vaguest notions of effectiveness and efficiency. Such groups are not easily managed, and with the stenos being paid by the week, productivity is haphazard.

In recent years, there has been a trend to outsource medical stenography to foreign contractors, particularly in India, where English is widely spoken, qualified people are willing to get themselves certified to U.S. standards, contractors are willing to conform to HIPAA requirements, and the Internet takes care of communications. Oh, and labor rates are low.

There are also onshore contractors who do the same, the only difference being that the stenos are (or are said to be) operating locally.

Some hospitals have dispersed their medical steno pools and now contract with the same stenos on a work-at-home basis.

All of these arrangements seem to work.

What are the common elements?

1. Pay is on a piecework basis.

2. There are contractual turnaround times.

3. Quality standards are enforced by contract (no meet, no pay).

Even if the stenographer in Coimbatore is being paid a dollar an hour, by the time various middlemen are paid, the actual net labor cost is not all that much lower than in-house stenographers. Lower, yes, but greatly lower, not likely.

However, labor cost per se is not the management issue. The management issue is timely delivery of completed work. That's hard to get from an hourly labor force of largely fixed capacity. The stenographer's cost, in the hospital's scheme of things, is hardly even round-off. But, every day that the average medical record is waiting for completed stenography is a day added to the payment collection cycle, which is bad.

This goes to asset utilization and cycle time, with the asset being accounts receivable, much more than it does to cost.

Contract Requirements

Here are typical requirements for an idealized medical stenography service:

1. Next-morning delivery

2. Error-free stenography, 95 percent of all dictations

3. Next-morning delivery of corrected stenography

4. Near-real-time delivery on a premium-payment basis

The traditional standard for good medical stenography is one error per hundred words, but that standard is actually pretty loose, allowing five errors per page. One error in a dictation means another lap around the circuit, so the appropriate measure is the fraction of dictations that need to make that second lap at all. One error or 20 errors in a dictation come to the same thing, one more lap.

Contractor Selection

With the contract requirements in hand, bids can be solicited from qualified contractors, including local, national, and worldwide.
Bids can be taken from the in-house stenography department.
Bids can be taken from a spun-off version of the in-house stenography department.

Implementation

Somebody has to be in charge of this service, and it is likely to require more than just commercial administration in the purchasing department. A manager is required.
That manager can track and evaluate.

BACK TO MAKE VERSUS BUY

At this point, with performance requirements supported by commercial terms in the contract, with a manager identified who is responsible for performance, and with tracking of performance established, it doesn't matter whether the supplier is an in-house group or an outside contractor.

Indeed, since the net labor cost savings is probably small, the make versus buy exercise is valid if it results in established performance standards for the in-house group, getting lethargy out of the old system, and getting vitality in.

Here are baseline questions to pose:

1. Is the backlog growing? (If not, then there is adequate capacity.)

2. Is the first draft being produced well ahead of the target delivery hour?

3. Is the proofreading being done well ahead of the target delivery hour?

4. Is there a valid internal quality evaluation system actually being applied, with periodic and episodic retraining?

5. Is anonymous tracking and posting of error rates being done?

6. Are post-proofreading errors being studied in each case? (These should be so rare as to cause alarm each time they occur.)

Backlogs are commonly used as a measure of overloading of any such department. However, if the backlog is not growing, then there is an *inventory* problem but not a *capacity* problem. Farm out the present inventory and then keep up with all new work. The backlog will not reoccur unless the workload expands beyond present capacity.

In most work groups, there is a tendency to slow down if the backlog is low, stretching the work. That's bad, and management needs to preclude that as an issue by establishing internal turnaround standards, so that it makes no difference to the worker whether there is a backlog or not. Piecework payment is another solution, but piecework compensation for in-house employees tends to be hard to administer. For at-home workers and outside contractors, piecework payment is fine.

GENERALIZING

Medical transcription service is used here as an example that every reader can follow. The same logic applies to every service department and function within the institution. The same make-or-buy conceptual process can lead to the establishment of performance standards, appropriate productivity, built-in training/retraining, and support of global (not local!) optimization.

17
Effectiveness versus Efficiency

The goal is to promote effective use of resources for the benefit of the patient. Efficiency comes as a result of effectiveness and should not be pursued separately.

CHECKLIST

☑ Effectiveness is to be measured against the global objective of serving the patient.

☑ Effectiveness trumps efficiency.

☑ Become effective first, then find ways to be efficient while retaining effectiveness.

EFFECTIVENESS FIRST

Let's consider supply problems. A nurse needs particular supplies to care for a patient. Suppose the supplies aren't there. Will the nurse write a memo? More likely, the nurse will see this as an obstacle to overcome, take action, and solve that particular supply problem as quickly as possible so that care can be provided to the patient. This is in fact part of the nursing culture, doing what's necessary to care for the patient. It's a fine thing.

This results in a point-solution, one that overcomes the specific problem in a local, limited way. On its own, this does not result in a general solution nor preclude the same problem from arising again and again.

Ad hoc solutions to supply problems are apt to move the problem (borrowing from the neighboring unit) rather than solving the problem. That is to say, a local solution is found, not a global solution.

Ad hoc solutions put a premium on informality.

Ad hoc solutions are rarely self-documenting and, indeed, may be intentionally nondocumenting. Raiding the supply cabinet in the next unit is an example.

Not all problems merit a general solution, and for some, informal *ad hoc* solutions may be the right answer. That should be a management policy decision, however, not a default condition.

HOARDING AS GOOD PRACTICE

Hoarding is *effective,* since most participants learn to be good hoarders, but it is not *efficient* because the hoarded inventory is off the books and may or may not be well deployed.

Several possible solutions arise:

- Leave the situation alone.

- Issue more and more supplies until even the least adept hoarders have plenty.

- Create an alternative solution that is both effective and efficient.

Management should be humble enough to recognize that no 'scientific management' solution may exist that is both as effective as the hoarding system in place and more efficient at the same time. Learned studies don't always reach this commonsense solution for lack of understanding the utter need to keep patient care going (Tucker 2003).

One management method now popular is 'lean operations management,' which will be covered in the next chapter. Caution: naïve application of lean operations management usually makes inventory control and deployment worse.

18

Lean Operations

"Lean" operations that reduce cycle time are fine and are integral to Six Sigma. "Lean" operations aimed at inventory and stocking-level control usually make things worse.

CHECKLIST

☑ Focus on cycle time.

☑ Be cautious in reducing stocking levels.

☑ Replenishment variability drives stocking levels up.

CYCLE TIME

The principles of cycle time management have been presented earlier in the book. They are summarized in Table 18.1.

NAÏVE LEAN INVENTORY 'MANAGEMENT'

Lean inventory strategies are intended to improve the balance sheet by reducing inventory.

Table 18.1   Topics related to cycle time.

Topic	Reference page
Know the bottleneck(s)	73
Schedule accordingly	43, 51, 61
Optimize globally, not locally	83
Defend in depth	129

They often rely on small-batch operations, pull-scheduling, and Machiavellian operations management.

The conceptual starting point is that productive units are hoarding inventory. The basic management method for finding the culprits is to 'starve the line' to find out who runs out of inventory last (!) Fine for Machiavelli, not so good for harmony in the workplace.

There are somewhat more polite ways to do this: by hectoring from above, by centralizing authority, by issuing memos. These rarely do any good, because responsible local managers and professionals in healthcare are going to make as sure as they can that they don't run out of supplies (page 113) and put their patients at risk.

PROPER LEAN INVENTORY ANALYSIS

To perform a proper lean inventory analysis, start with the 'safety stocking level,' which is the predetermined minimum level for a stocked item at the point of use. That's the number of items that might be required suddenly, on an unscheduled basis, plus a little bit more. This is the absolute minimum. The actual level should never, ever fall below this level. That's why it's called the safety level.

Note that the safety stocking level is set by local management, not by the purchasing department. The safety stocking level, if all cards are on the table, includes the hoarding level.

Next, consider the reorder level and the replenishment time.

Calculate the rate of consumption of the item. If it is variable, calculate on the high side.

Determine the time required to replenish, including internal paperwork. How many hours or days to restock? If it is variable, figure on the high side.

Calculate the number of items, conservatively, that can be consumed during the time it takes to replenish the stock. That is, multiply the consumption rate per hour by the replenishment time duration in hours.

That's the nominal replenishment order quantity.

Add the nominal replenishment order quantity to the safety stock level. That sum is the reordering level.

Local management orders up a replenishment quantity when the local stock level falls near the reordering level. See Figure 18.1.

The supply department replenishes on demand (pull-management of local inventory resupply). The supply department may wish to deliver even more product just to reduce the number of trips, which is okay but does not go in the direction of leanness.

So far, no consideration has been given to delays or upsets. This is a nice copybook exercise, so far, but not of much value in the real world.

REAL-LIFE SUPPLY MANAGEMENT

The point of Six Sigma is to optimize in favor of the patient, which in this case means, don't run out of supplies. Therefore, the essential

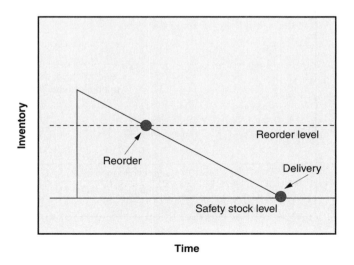

Figure 18.1   Ideal inventory levels.

supply management activity is to focus on reliability and timeliness of replenishment. These combine into one factor, the variability of replenishment time. The reorder level should be the safety stocking level plus the number of items, with 95 percent confidence, that will be consumed by the time the replenishment is accomplished. The 95 percent level is equal to the average replenishment time plus two standard deviations of the replenishment time, based on historical experience. Working on variability gives twice the leverage as working on the mean value itself.

Moreover, the safety stock is also determined in real life by the variability in the replenishment time, because local management expresses its lack of confidence in timely replenishment by driving up the safety stocking level.

The variability of replenishment time, like all variabilities, includes controllable and noncontrollable variability. Get to work on the controllable variabilities. Consider trade-offs. For instance, it may be good strategy to pay a small premium in unit price to get more reliable replenishment times.

Figure 18.2 shows that the variability of replenishment time drives up the peak, average, and minimum inventory levels. The

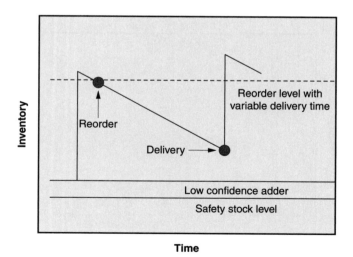

Figure 18.2 Real-world inventory levels.

variability in the replenishment time shows up directly as a financial burden on the institution.

Therefore, there is substantial financial, as well as operational, incentive to reduce the variability in replenishment time for all products.

The modern way to reduce the inventory level on the balance sheet is to order smaller quantities, more often. That's a good idea if the variability is zero. But, if the variability is not zero, then the inventory level stays high on its own. So, get the variability under control first, then move toward smaller batches.

Stock-Out Consequences

In a factory, if a local production unit runs out of inventory, production halts for a period of time. This has some economic consequence, which can be figured out in a trade-off analysis of lost or delayed production versus reduced work-in-progress inventory.

In a hospital, the consequences might be a good deal more severe. Safety stock means *safety* stock.

When the Patient Is the Inventory

Scheduling patient treatment has been discussed in earlier chapters (see chapters 6, 8, and 9, pages 43, 51, and 61), where the evaluation dealt with patient convenience and productivity.

Hoarding

Hoarding is an expression of lack of confidence in the replenishment system. It is not only natural, it is prudent. (Cf. page 85 above).

The only way to reduce hoarding is to persuade the local unit managers that resupply is trustworthy. That's a long slog, because the natural tendency is to remember that one time when . . . .

Tracking charts and proven performance may eventually win over the hoarders. That's okay. Patient protection, patient care, and patient service are all more important than the balance sheet.

Lets consider wheelchairs as an example. Wheelchairs are never where they are needed, they are always where they were needed last. Wheelchairs are expensive, patients steal them, they get beat up, and they are conspicuous when sitting around idle, so the natural tendency is to believe that there are too many of them.

So what does responsible local unit management do? Hoard wheelchairs.

Wheelchairs are not consumed, other than by theft and casualty loss, so the purchasing/central stores/supply chain model discussed earlier does not quite apply. The arithmetic does though. For each patient care unit there is some safety stocking level of wheelchairs, which is at least one wheelchair and probably more. There is a consumption rate of wheelchairs, which each unit can determine from experience. There is also a spontaneous generation level of wheelchairs, which are the ones that come in from other departments and get left behind.

So, wheelchairs move around, depleted in one place and piling up in another. How can management possibly figure out whether the total number of wheelchairs is correct? Are there too many wheelchairs for the actual need? Should each department have its own color-coded wheelchairs, and would that mean a higher total count or a lower one? Even if it were higher, would that make the problem go away?

Yipes!

Every supermarket has figured this out. A supermarket needs as many shopping carts as the peak number of shoppers plus the number of carts in the parking lot corrals.

The supermarket does not want to reduce the number of shoppers, certainly not by making them wait for a shopping cart, so customer service determines the supermarket's safety stocking level for shopping carts, never to be violated.

The number of shopping carts sitting in the parking lot corrals is determined entirely by the number of cart wranglers the supermarket employs to fetch the carts back into the store. In addition, there are always a few scattered here and there, and some few shoppers steal shopping carts.

Supermarket management can do a simple trade-off: number of shopping carts owned (inventory) versus number of wranglers employed (labor cost).

The same applies to wheelchairs in hospitals.

The safety stock level for the whole of the hospital is the sum of the unit safety stock levels. The net consumption rate in each unit can be estimated, and it may be positive or negative for various times of the day.

The number of wheelchairs that are in the equivalent of the supermarket parking lot corrals (overstocked care units) is determined by the number of wheelchair wranglers employed.

Should nurses, X-ray technicians, orderlies, and other professionals and paraprofessionals be used as wheelchair wranglers? Maybe. It would be an interesting management exercise to figure this one out.

The starting and ending point, though, is to make sure that every unit always has its safety stock level of wheelchairs, even if by hoarding. When local unit managers develop a high level of trust in the wrangler–replenishment system, then the hoarding levels will go down over time.

Tracking charts of stock level for each unit help build that level of trust.

For further information on Six Sigma methods and tools, see page 161.

Systems

19

Six Sigma Design Principles

There are design principles for producing trustworthy systems. These are distilled from centuries of experience and can be applied directly to healthcare, manual operations included.

CHECKLIST

☑ Select the preferred method.

☑ Do it the same way every time.

☑ Track attainment.

☑ Two birds, two stones.

☑ Target the center of the range.

☑ Defend the patient in depth.

WHAT'S DIFFERENT ABOUT A SIX SIGMA DESIGN?

Six Sigma, while seeking very high goals, is a very cautious package of practices. The Six Sigma design rules, which follow, are very simple.

1. *Select the preferred method.* Well, why would a nonpreferred method be chosen? Would that make any sense? This has been discussed extensively, page 11, in choosing protocols based on national standards.

2. *Do it the same way every time.* This consistency reduces controllable variability and conforms to common sense. Note that this discourages experimentation and freelancing, even if done with the best of intentions and intuition. Experiment off-line.

3. *Track attainment.* Keep score. Post the scores. Tracking attainment informs and reinforces the progress already made.

4. *Two birds, two stones.* Subdivide tasks, if necessary, for the good reason that one task cannot serve two masters. Here's a small example. The chief nursing officer[1] of a large hospital found that in one patient care department the several nurses all had the right to open the departmental narcotics safe but there was only one key, which was carried by the last nurse to have opened the safe. The next nurse who wanted access had to find the prior nurse, which wasted time and energy. The hospital was a research hospital, so a study was performed to determine the number of wasted minutes per shift per nurse. Using that lost-production fact, the chief nursing officer was able to get more keys and issue them, one to each nurse.

Okay, but why do you suppose the number of keys had been severely limited in the first place? Surely for narcotics loss control. If lots of keys are in circulation, what's the mechanism for narcotics loss control? The one-key design had two outputs but only paid heed to one of them. The many-key design has two outputs but only pays heed to the other of them. What's needed is something more; the task needs to be subdivided so that both outputs can be given heed. That 'something more' may result in higher cost or some other burden, but that's not an excuse to do nothing or to pretend that one stone is going to hit two birds very often.

5. *Target the center of the range.* Targeting the center of the range discourages taking 'just barely' as a satisfactory result. It may be

---

1. Personal communication, although the story has been presented at conferences.

'satisfactory' for this one instance, but in a larger system, if all tasks were done just barely, the likelihood of overall success would vaporize. This is self-evident, is it not? Yet it is considered one of the essential reasons for the success of Japanese manufacturing companies after World War II. American manufacturing in those days was based on go/no-go acceptance, which always degenerates to just-barely. That's why Japanese car doors slammed well and American car doors did not, among other things.

6. *Defend the patient in depth.* See page 129. Protecting the patient is not only a good idea, there are systematic ways to improve the likelihood that it will occur.

EFFECTIVENESS

Six Sigma goes for effectiveness, high attainment, and safe patients. This will very likely lead to high utilization of resources and, thereby, provide efficient operations. Trying to improve utilization by going at this the other way around, by reducing costs, is not apt to work. Effectiveness first, efficiency second.

In other words, reduce cost but only by selecting between effective solutions. Take the least-cost *effective* solution. Just make sure it's really a solution.

20
Defense in Depth

Because errors and mistakes cannot be excluded, particularly in manual operations, the patient must be protected in depth from any hazard.

CHECKLIST

☑ No failure from this point forward will put the patient at risk.

☑ Validate inputs.

☑ Take stock before taking irreversible steps.

THIS POINT FORWARD

The whole point of *defense in depth* is that no single, credible failure from this point forward will put the patient at risk.

With human beings involved, there is no way to preclude single, credible failures, and so the system design itself must tolerate such failures without putting the patient at risk.

The way to consider this systematically is to lay out all the steps in sequence on a flowchart (see page 177).

Start with the *last* flowchart box. At that last box, the design must be such that any credible, single failure will not harm the patient.

Back up one box on the flowchart. Identify all the things that can credibly go wrong, one at a time. Make sure, considering this box and the final box, no credible single failure can harm the patient.

Repeat with the preceding box, always considering all implications from that box forward.

Walk all the way back to the first box.

Think about the information flow. Each stage has the following elements:

Decision → Action → Evidence

Let's walk this backward and ask:

1. What evidence is needed to determine if the action was completed properly or not?

2. What information is produced by the action itself, while the action is going on?

3. What information does the person making the decision require?

A well-designed stage produces clear evidence regarding the outcome, the action itself produces clear information as the process is going on, and the decision to proceed to do the action is based on clear information available at that time.

To the extent that the element is weak on any of these, trouble lurks.

For instance, suppose the action is to give a verbal instruction. What evidence will there be that the instruction was both received and understood? Industry standards now call for certain instructions to be read back, and that's fine. How about all those other verbal instructions, shouldn't they be repeated back, too?

The linkage to prior stages, as we are walking backward, is through the decision. Part of the necessary information to enable the decision is the evidence from upstream stages. Indeed, the necessary information for each stage determines the evidence requirement for the stage or stages immediately upstream.

This is repeated, stage by stage, walking backward.

LOOKING UPSTREAM

Looking upstream from any box on the flowchart, failures that may already have happened must be spotted and tied off.

Since upstream failures cannot be excluded, the system needs to have ways of detecting existing failures and precluding latent (undetected) failures.

This is done by validating the inputs to each box. This is a familiar notion, since second diagnoses are standard medical practice. It is also standard medical practice to have two professionals calculating drug doses at bedside. Pharmacists cross-check medicine orders against prior medicine orders for the same patient to check for contraindications.

Let's call that extra protective action a *gate*. See page 151. A *gate* is a second, independent action intended to validate an input. Until validated, the gate stays closed. When validated, the gate opens and the process continues.

The gate need not always be a repetition by an equal practitioner. It may be a simple clipboard checkoff and inspection. Common sense applies.

POINT OF NO RETURN

Just before each irreversible action, put in a time buffer to allow time to take stock, review the validity of all inputs, and review the actions to be taken in the next few steps.

Stop, look around. Take stock.

It is now recommended practice to do this just before the first surgical incision to reduce the likelihood of being at the wrong site. How can surgery happen at the wrong site? By having an undetected upstream error. It is common practice now for the surgeon to mark the site in person well before the patient is draped for surgery. That's good. The flowchart box upstream of this? How does the surgeon find out where the site is supposed to be? Where's the gate?

Some institutions have two people mark the site beforehand. That provides a gate, but do both of those marker people get their input from a single source? Where are the two gates? Some ask the patient to mark the site. Is the patient to be trusted? Concerned, yes; but trusted?

THE PRINCIPLE OF OPTIMALITY

There is an entire area of mathematics that deals with optimum paths. *Optimum* in our case means treating the necessity for patient safety as a constraint on the choices and actions to be taken, and then figuring out the preferred way to proceed while respecting this constraint.

There is a principle of optimality known as Bellman's principle, which is wonderfully terse and easy to understand:

The optimum path is composed of optimum segments (Bellman 1957).

Bellman provides a modicum of comfort by assuring that since each of these path segments is optimum, then the whole path is optimum. That may not in its own be a really strong reason to do it this way, but it does reinforce common sense.

Application of Bellman's principle is almost always backward-marching, as it is applied here.

INNOCENT INTERFERENCE

One special factor intrudes in designing systems for healthcare. Patients and family may interfere with equipment if there is anything within reach. To take two examples from author Smith's nursing experience: parents in a pediatric unit pull off EKG electrical leads to see how long it takes a nurse to get to the bed. What's more, patients and family respond to the beeper on an IV by twisting any knobs within reach. This is anticipated in IV equipment design by providing a lock-out device for the nurse to use to defeat any such disruptive actions.

Healthcare systems need to contemplate this innocent yet hazardous phenomenon.

FAILURE MODES AND EFFECTS

Now we can look at the classical failure modes and their effects.

For each stage, what failure modes are possible (not necessarily likely, but possible)?

Which of these will be disregarded because the trust level is high?

Of those remaining, taken one at a time, which ones put the patient in harm's way? If any do, what changes are necessary to provide an additional layer of protection for the patient?

The changes may be a different sequencing of events, they may be the insertion of additional inspections, they may be a redesign of the action entirely.

For instance, there are said to be 800,000 sharps events each year reported to OSHA (HHS 1998). There are OSHA-mandated receptacles for needles used in hospitals, and however many such receptacles are provided, they never seem to be in the right place. What additional layers of protection could be provided that would satisfy sterility requirements, convenience (likelihood of actually being used), and practicality for syringes and suture needles? Some have suggested providing a cork to jab the needle into, protecting patient and nurse as well, until the needle gets into the receptacle. What would be a better idea?

CRITICAL ITEMS LIST

Combining the items that are considered trustworthy and the failure modes and effects, makes a critical items list. Assign priority to changes to be made.

It's good practice to update the critical items list as the analysis is going on, so that items identified early on don't get lost in the shuffle.

THE MARCH OF TIME

Rushing things doesn't help. With so many manual operations and so many decisions to be made in even simple processes, wisdom lies in providing time for each task to be done and results to be confirmed. Building-in pauses so that stock can be taken is prudent, particularly just before irreversible actions.

Emphasis must be on getting it right, checking all along the way, fixing little things that need to be fixed, and proceeding.

The way to get things done more quickly is not to rush; it is to redesign the process so that each step has a very high likelihood of being done right the first time.

TOOL KIT

Table 20.1 lists tools that are often helpful in evaluating existing processes and designing new ones.

BLAME-FREE WORKPLACE

The workplace environment must encourage people who detect errors to declare the error, even if it is their own error, rather than covering it up or pretending it didn't happen. While this is self-evident, it is not a natural course of human behavior. To get this to work consistently, the workplace must be blame-free (Juran 1995, Aguayo 1990).

This applies to persons who flag a departure from normal, too. This is called *stopping the line.* Should everybody be authorized to

Table 20.1 Tools for the tool kit.

Topic	Page
Process flowcharts	177
Task design	147
System design	125
Failure modes and effects	133
Chains of events	183
Three-plane perspective	185
Robust communications	137

stop the line? After all, the person raising the flag may be mistaken, perhaps there is nothing wrong. Should the most junior person in the group be authorized to stop the line? The textbook answer is yes, but it's not easy to achieve in the real world. If the flag-raiser is rewarded with a scolding, don't expect any flag-raising in the future, from this person or any other.

A blame-free workplace is one in which it is acknowledged that human beings make inadvertent errors and that the proper and effective corrective action is to retrain the person so that the likelihood of repetition is low. A retraining support system is required. A management culture that resists the temptation to blame is required. This takes work. Management work, because management sets the tone.

An error-cognizant system has the following features:

- The possibility of inadvertent error is acknowledged.

- Errors are detected before harm is done.

- Single errors can do no harm to a patient, by design.

- Humans who make inadvertent errors are retrained, not blamed.

We admit that some small number of humans make malicious errors. Any such persons need to be identified and excluded. Defense in depth and a blame-free environment deal well with inadvertent error but not with malicious error. It is surpassingly difficult to design against malicious error.

21

Communications Systems Design

Robust communications include confirmation that the message got through and was understood.

CHECKLIST

☑ The responsible party is identified beforehand.

☑ A trustworthy communications medium is used.

☑ The loop is closed.

A STARTING POINT

The *Wall Street Journal*, April 9, 2004, front page, reported, "Many U.S. adults risk medical errors because they don't comprehend terminology used by doctors and insurers, the Institute of Medicine said."

GENERAL MODEL

Let's start with the diagram in Figure 21.1.

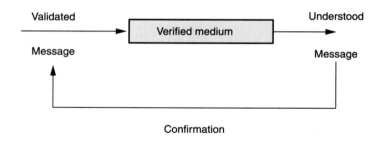

Figure 21.1 Ingredients essential to communications.

Somebody has to be in charge. Somebody has to be responsible to see that the communications got through and got understood. That's almost always the sender.

Considering the quotation from the *Wall Street Journal,* when a physician speaks to a patient, which party is the more responsible? The patient is the one with the keen interest, so there is a case to be made that the patient is the one to be held responsible. On the other hand, the physician is the one who has the information to be imparted. How do you vote?

Being responsible for your own healthcare is a popular theme these days, but when it gets down to a specific message to be communicated from doctor to patient, we believe that the doctor has to be the responsible party.

The doctor, being responsible, needs to see that the message got through and was understood. This means more than getting a release signed by the patient, it means interrogating the patient and taking note of the responses.

The same applies to every caregiver dealing with a patient and/or family member.

This takes time and effort. It's worth it.

Note that the *Wall Street Journal* doesn't say patients don't understand the words doctors say. It says patients don't understand the message. The message may be spoken, it may be written. There may be any number of language problems, and not just Latin.

A lesson may be learned from the instruction sheets that come with consumer products these days, which are often picture stories with little in the way of text. That's good. They bypass language difficulties and paint a picture better than any written or spoken text could ever do. The instruction sheets also provide a toll-free number to call for support. That's good, too. These lessons can be applied, and sometimes are, to medical instructions. Yet even with pictures, it is important that the doctor take the time to make sure that the patient got the message. Ditto for nurses or any other professionals who find themselves in this position.

PERSON TO PERSON—VERBAL COMMUNICATIONS

Many healthcare communications are verbal from one caregiver to another. Some of these have life and death implications. Time may be of the essence.

Closing the communications loop is nonetheless mandatory. Indeed, urgency and importance both militate for confirmation that the message was received and understood.

The centuries-old solution is for the receiver to repeat back the message. That's the way navies have done it, based on their own experience in noisy, frenetic, urgent circumstances. It's what we all do when we are given a telephone number over the telephone, we read it back to make sure. It's what we require children to do when instructions are given to them. It works. It takes very little time. It closes the loop.

Note that closing the loop deals with several points of potential failure. The sender may have misspoken, thinking A but saying B. When the loop is closed back to the sender, there is a reasonable chance that the failure will be recognized and corrected on the spot.

Suppose the message is lost in the noise. Then, the confirmation return message[1] asking for a repetition makes the failure evident.

Suppose the receiver hears B but misapprehends, thinking C. When C is said back to the sender, the failure is evident and can be corrected on the spot.

Suppose the receiver misspeaks and says back D. Again, the failure will be evident.

---

1. This is a negative acknowledgement in the communications world, NACK instead of ACK.

Closing the communications loop deals with all of these and is *required* if the communications are to be trustworthy. Saying back or reading back is now the standard for certain key communications in the healthcare professions. It should be practiced in all instances of verbal communications because there are few communications that do not have importance, eventually, to the patient.

THOSE ACRONYMS!

Let's deal with the many, many acronyms that shorten communications but have their own sort of failures. It's easy to misunderstand a string of spoken letters, particularly over the telephone.

This problem has a known solution, practiced by millions the world over every day. It's to use a set of carefully selected words to represent the alphabet. It's called a phonetic alphabet (see Figure 21.2).

Here's a simple example that does not involve the whole alphabet. Cable installers[2] use two kinds of fittings on the ends of the cables.

Alpha	Juliet	Sierra
Bravo	Kilo	Tango
Charlie	Lima	Uniform
Delta	Mike	Victor
Echo	November	Whiskey
Foxtrot	Oscar	X-ray
Golf	Papa	Yankee
Hotel	Quebec	Zebra
India	Romeo	

If you don't think Quebec has a *q* sound, say, "cucumber." Some say *Indiana* instead of *India,* for the cadence.

Figure 21.2   The phonetic alphabet.

---

2. This is drawn from author Barry's own experience.

One is called FC, the other SC. Try guessing which is being said, particularly over a telephone or walkie-talkie. No chance. So, cable installers don't say FC or SC, they say Frank-Charlie or Sam-Charlie. It's a great solution that works every time.

There are full phonetic alphabets. The most common one these days was developed by the U.S. military with careful attention to avoiding sounds that people with various mother tongues find difficult to say. There is almost no risk of any of these words being confused with any other. It's easy to learn and retain. Furthermore, only the speaker needs to know the phonetic alphabet, the listener can understand the meaning immediately with no training at all. Isn't that remarkable?

Digits are enunciated as: one, two, tree,[3] four, five, six, seven, eight'-er, nine'-er, and zero. Numbers are always read left to right, one at a time[4] as if reading a telephone number out loud. Do just a few, then pause.

These are most effective when done in a sing-song fashion to put extra emphasis on the accented syllables.

PERSON TO PERSON—HANDWRITTEN COMMUNICATIONS

Handwriting in the medical field is notoriously bad. Many believe that the billions of dollars being put into computerized physician's order systems provide only one benefit, the elimination of handwritten physician's orders. Nurse managers[5] report that professional hours are lost every day because physicians have to be chased down to have handwritten orders explained.

In other professions, an illegible note would bring obloquy upon the writer. But, sad to say, that doesn't apply to the medical field.

Refer back to the communications diagram in Figure 21.1 and the discussion of responsibility for the communication. Where is the confirmatory loop-closing? Who is responsible for the message getting

---

3. Yes, that's *tree*.

4. Seventy and seventeen are too difficult to disambiguate, to take one example.

5. This is drawn from author Smith's own experience.

through? Not for the message being scribbled on an order pad, but for getting through? Surely it is the sender.

Now, let's consider solutions. Computerized physician's order systems do not pretend to decode the physician's handwriting, but rather provide an alternative means for the physician to enter the order, picking order-items off menus and lists.

That same thing can be done with preprinted order pads and check-boxes. A preprinted form with a thousand check-boxes would not work, but how about two dozen? That would cover maybe 90 percent of the order-items, and blanks could be provided for the physician to write in, carefully, those less-often-called-for items.

Note that closing the loop is still required, even if the written message or computer-entered message or checked-off message is perfectly clear. The receiver needs to confirm back to sender that the message was received and understood. Otherwise, the responsible party, the sender, cannot know if the communication was completed. Responsibility abides with the sender.

PERSON TO MACHINE COMMUNICATIONS

It is believed that Chinese artisans discovered how to make porcelain in ancient times, and then they forgot how. It had to be relearned centuries later.

Come now to modern times. Four decades ago, information going into a computer was never, ever entered wrongly because the information was punched into a card and then repunched a second time on a second machine that compared the key stroke to the already-punched column on the card. The likelihood of both operations making the same mistake was very nearly zero.

That's been lost! Yipes! It's worse than garbage-in/garbage-out. Now with databases and linked applications, it's garbage-in/garbage-can't-get-it-out.

Most data-entry schemes today provide some shallow internal consistency, for example, checking that an entry in a zip code field has the right quantity of numerals, but few if any do more than that. Suppose a blood pressure is keyed in as 150/75 rather than 105/75. What internal checking is going to find that failure?

Data entry must be verified and validated.

The simplest way to verify is simply to enter the data twice. This takes very little time and eliminates key-entry mistakes. This requires that the data-entry software be capable of supporting this, but that's a trivial software programming task.

If double entry is not available, then the next option is to force the data entry person to accept/reject the data by showing small sets of the entered information back to the person in pop-up panes. This is not a high-value check because people tend not to find their own mistakes, but it works reasonably well if the check is done by a second person. Note that this takes more software design work than just entering everything twice in the first place.

It is common software design practice to force users to enter *some* data twice, such as passwords, when the significance of the particular datum is high. But in healthcare, when is the value of the data ever low?

It is common to use pop-up data confirmation panels, too, in like circumstances.

Since it is easier and faster to set things up so that they are simply entered twice in the first place, using the same double-entry policies that accountants have used for centuries, that's the way to go.

Double entry *verifies* the entries. That's not enough because the inputs may be invalid. In most cases, the key-entry person cannot know if the data are *valid,* nor can the computer, but validity checking can be applied to spot suspect information.

To be of any value, the validity checking must be deep. Counting the number of digits entered for a zip code is not deep enough. Checking the entered zip code against the street address and telephone area code is better. Looking up the subscriber's name for the offered telephone number helps. Tests such as these require only Internet access these days plus a modest programming effort.

Validity of observed data can be checked for consistency. If the patient's blood pressure is entered, then a tracking chart should be popped up so that the data entry person can spot suspect data if only because it is not consistent with prior data. This won't catch 125 in place of 123, but it will likely call attention to 105 in place of 150.

Consider computerized physician's order entry systems, which present a list of drug order options, hundreds of them. Given that

list-picking with a stylus or mouse is error-prone, what levels of protection should the software provide? Should the software insist on
being fed the diagnosis, patient characteristics, and allergies first, so
that only those drug order options that are conventional are even
shown to the doctor, subject to some override facility so that the
doctor can cope with an unusual patient need? That would reduce
the opportunity for inadvertent error in the first place, which is
easier and better than chasing down order-entry errors later on.

Standardized protocols and care plans, page 14, go in the right
direction and can be supported by software that presents the doctor
with the standard options first.

MACHINE TO MACHINE COMMUNICATIONS

Machine to machine communications these days close the loop and do
even more, adding check data into the message stream. The machines
report any discrepancy and even keep logs for review later on. So
failures in machine to machine communications are negligible.

What is still worth some consideration, though, is the display of
status by machines, particularly linked machines. It's good practice
for the machines to declare what they are doing, starting with the fact
that they are alive (using a 'heartbeat' indicator) and doing task X or
doing task Y. The machines themselves don't care, but humans in the
neighborhood, particularly those who are relying on these machines,
could take some comfort.

MACHINE TO PERSON COMMUNICATIONS

The person using a machine needs to be trained to understand the
machine.

That training needs to cover both normal and off-normal operations.

Information overload needs to be eliminated by design of the
machine-to-person interface. *Information*, used here in the narrowest
sense, is that which could not have been predicted. So, the number

on the next toss of the dice is, when the dice are tossed, *information*. A computer display can have lots and lots of data on a screen and have no *information* at all, if all those data are routine values.

People can cope with only a few pieces of information at a time, and then only rather slowly. A common blunder in computer display design is to overwhelm the person with information by triggering too many notices, error messages, or alarms all at once. This presents the person with an unreasonable burden.

Second, machines need to eliminate ambiguity and provide a margin against ambiguity. Consider the common X-ray film. At a glance, it is not obvious whether the film is being viewed from the front or from the back, and every healthcare professional seems to have had a personal experience where something awful almost happened because the X-ray film was in the viewer backward. There is not enough margin against ambiguity, even though it would be trivial to tell the film supplier to make one side a different color. There is usually a number printed on the front face of the film, which is a step in the right direction; however, for most X-ray machines, that number is not printed on the film by the camera but by a different machine. The technician takes the film out of the camera and puts it into the number-writer. If the technician inadvertently turns the film over . . . . Where is the defensive margin against this?

There are plenty of examples of weak machine design in healthcare, and it's something the industry has to clean up in the next generation, with much better input from the machine-using community. It's not trivial, it takes lots of careful thought, and it has to be done.

22

Tasks

There are three rules for effective task design: make the task more likely to produce the right result than the wrong one, make it possible to detect error on the spot, and make it possible to correct any error on the spot.

CHECKLIST

☑ The task needs to have a better chance of producing the right result than a wrong one.

☑ Errors need to be evident on the spot.

☑ Means to correct the error on the spot need to be provided.

☑ Learn from experience.

POKA YOKE

The first three of these have one of those cute Japanese names. This one is *poka yoke,* which is pronounced as the first half of *Pocahontas* followed by *okay*[1] with a *y* in front of it. The authors are

---

1. This is sometimes heard as 'yolk.' The Japanese pronunciation is somewhere in between.

advised[2] that this is Japanese slang, that there is no way to write it in the classical Japanese ideographs. It means 'prevention of inadvertent error' (Barry 2002, 19).

Note that it does not mean prevention of malicious error, thoughtless error, or foolish error. It means prevention of inadvertent error.

The starting point is a belief that while all workers make an inadvertent error from time to time, there is no reason to believe that the error was intentional, foolish, or inattentive. If an error happens inadvertently, then fix it. Maybe retrain the worker, but don't get judgmental about it. A blame-free workplace is what everybody should want.

After all, the person making the next inadvertent error might be . . . .

First Poka Yoke Rule

Make the right outcome more likely than a wrong one. Training is one part of this. So is designing the task itself so that a normal human being can do it reliably. Provide tooling where that is possible, although for lots of the manual operations in healthcare, the prospect is not bright.

Consider kits, interlocks, color-coded parts, warning lights, left-handed layouts for southpaws,[3] check-off lists, and so on (Barry 2002, 21).

Allow plenty of time for neophytes to complete the task. Speed comes with mastery.

Second Poka Yoke Rule

Errors need to be obvious, on the spot. This is not easy to achieve in many cases, since tasks are sometimes done by feel, out of sight. Still, the rule is a good one.

Consider the classic case of leaving a sponge behind after surgery. If the sponge were evident, it would not be left behind. But

---

2. Personal communication, Prof. Dr. Tatsuo Iwamori, Tokyo Denki University.

3. Many left-handed people cannot use left-handed tools such as left-handed scissors, because they have been acculturated into the right-handed world. Left-handed layout helps, though.

if the sponge is out of sight, then the error is not obvious. Counting doesn't seem to be enough.

There is new technology that helps by putting a radio tag on every sponge, with the tag being readable, by radio, inexpensively, from outside the body (Roebuck 2004). Appendix E, page 231, addresses this very poka yoke rule.

So, to take the lesson, look for additional instrumentation to get this rule to work.

Third Poka Yoke Rule

Fix it on the spot—this implies that each task be broken down into small bites so that fixing it can be a meaningful concept. It is self-evident that fixing the error on the spot saves time and bother compared to fixing it any time later.

Fixing it on the spot, particularly if the fix is done by the worker *pro se*, gets the worker's attention spontaneously and should go in the direction of better results next time.

Poka Yoke Is Prudent

It is prudent to figure that inadvertent errors will come to pass. It is rash to think they will not.

Starting with that point of view, designing each task with the poka yoke rules in mind gives the best chance that the outcome will be the correct one, that latent errors will not be passed along to the next stage, and that overall system performance will be pleasing. In particular, this means designing any new task or redesigning any old task so that information will be available to act on.

Poka Yoke and Tracking Charts

If things that go wrong are fixed on the spot, then it is not likely that reports will be generated and attention paid. There is no built-in learning process[4] other than perhaps for the particular worker or those close at hand.

---

4. This was considered earlier in this book, see page 114, and elsewhere (Tucker 2003).

It would be nice to gather some data on the frequency of errors, even of errors corrected on the spot, for a particular task so that there is an informed basis for considering redesign of the task, the training, or the whole process. Tracking charts will serve. They take some additional bother, so there is no point in pretending that errors for every task will be tracked. Rather, encourage groups or work teams to pick their pet peeve and track that. Not only will the data be generated, but the incremental attention being paid may lead to a handy change in the task that takes the peevishness away.

23

Gates

Gates are points in the process that stop action until upstream conditions are validated. Gates block the propagation of error.

CHECKLIST

☑ Pick an activity, a block on a flowchart.

☑ Identify the at-risk inputs from upstream.

☑ Put a gate on each of those.

GATES

A gate prevents errors from propagating. Gates are, at a minimum, to be placed upstream of irreversible actions. The arithmetic is persuasive, as can be seen in Figure 23.1.

Stated somewhat differently, if the upstream action has a one percent error rate, a gate with 95 percent reliability will catch 19 out of 20 of those errors, so that only one out of 2000 (five out of 10,000) errors gets through to the next stage. That's a 20-fold improvement.

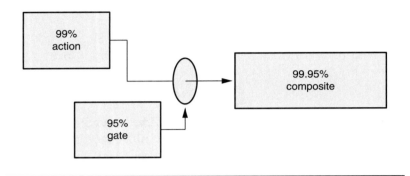

Figure 23.1   Gates to improve reliability.

Note that in this example, the gate itself is less reliable than the action. It is the combination of two fairly reliable, independent elements that gives a very reliable outcome. If a second independent gate were applied, then the composite error rate would drop by another factor. For instance, if a second independent gate of 95% reliability is added, the composite error rate would drop from one in 2000 to one in 40,000.

The key to getting this to work is to have independence between the upstream action and the gate or gates.

Suppose the upstream action is the physician's diagnosis. Suppose the gate is a second opinion. That should be independent.

Suppose the upstream action is a nurse's calculation of a drug dose based on the patient's body weight. Suppose that the gate is the same calculation done by a second nurse. That should be independent.

Now suppose that the first nurse declares, "I calculate 20,000 units," in the hearing of the second nurse. Or suppose that a physician does the first calculation and a nurse does the second. Will the nurse be independent or will the nurse be intimidated by what the doctor declares?

Often, the gate will be an inspection rather than a duplicate action. It's good if the inspection has some technology supporting it. Consider, for instance, the age-old issue of figuring out if all the sponges have been removed after surgery. Counting the sponges is an inspection step. As mentioned in Chapter 22 and Appendix E, a nurse has recently patented the use of tiny, inexpensive radio computer chips fixed to each sponge (Roebuck 2004). Since the RFID[1] chip reports its serial number when interrogated by a wand, even through the skin, the inspection step accounts for every sponge by serial number, in the body or in the disposal bin. That's a big improvement in gate reliability.

If the gate is a manual inspection, then the inspection should be done from a check-off list, the same way pilots and copilots do it before every take-off. This is particularly necessary if a person is checking his or her own work.

---

1. See Appendix E, page 231 for more information and other applications.

24

Buffers

Buffers are waiting times built into processes just upstream of irreversible actions to provide time to take stock.

CHECKLIST

☑ Identify key stages, those that are irreversible, really expensive, or uncomfortable for the patient.

☑ Put a buffer just upstream of each such stage.

☑ Use the buffer to take stock before proceeding.

BUFFERS

A *buffer* is a hold point, an intentional pause, inserted at key points in a process. The purpose is to allow all parties to confirm status and to reconfirm the plan for the subsequent step. See Figure 24.1 for an illustration.

It has become common practice to insert a buffer into surgical procedures to allow for reconfirmation of the surgical site.

The same logic applies to the launch point of any irreversible action, and it applies to the launch point of any action involving

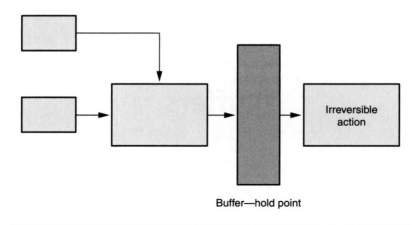

Buffer—hold point

Figure 24.1 Buffers to improve reliability.

several people. "Okay, team. We're going to lift the patient by lifting up on the blanket, and we are going to move the patient to this stretcher. Fred will hold the patient's head. On the count of three. Are we ready?" Restating the obvious is a good thing to do, for the same reason that pilots and copilots run through the preflight inspection even if they fly the same plane every day and make six takeoffs a day. It doesn't hurt, and it might help.

25
Centrality

Six Sigma does not accept go/no-go system design, but rather insists on targeting the center of the target range.

CHECKLIST

☑ Establish the nominal target as well as the tolerable range.

☑ Aim for the nominal target.

☑ Use go/no-go for rejection, but not for targeting.

TARGET THE CENTER OF THE RANGE

If two or three subsystems are meeting their specified ranges, but just barely so, then the larger system is going to be on the ragged edge all the time. It is not enough that each subsystem meets a go/no-go test or a pass/fail test; it is important that the distribution of the outcomes of each subsystem be well centered within the specified range. This contribution to robust system design is generally ascribed to Genichi Taguchi and is quite different from traditional American design practice, which was most often go/no-go (Taguchi 1999).

One way to promote central targeting is to provide a weighted scoring system that gives a higher score if the result is near the middle of the specified range. One popular scoring system uses a curve such the one in Figure 25.1. This one uses a weight that varies with the square of the distance from the central target. This process is often called *mean-square weighting*.

A centered distribution, as in the lower left diagram of Figure 25.1, gets a high score. Skewed distributions, such as those in the lower center and lower right positions, get progressively lower scores as the skew becomes more pronounced. Skewed distributions invite difficulties, and this is an easy and straightforward way of calling attention to the skew.

Target the center. Look for a high score. If the score goes down, look to see what's going on.

Numerical scoring is fine if the data are in a computer. If not, an estimate by eye is still quite helpful.

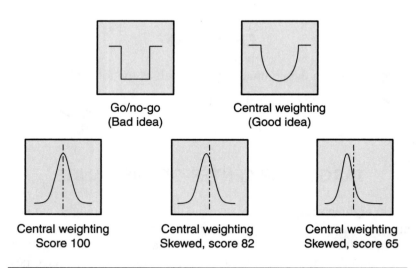

Figure 25.1 Centrality measures.

SEPARATE CONTROL FROM PROTECTION

If the result of a task is outside the tolerable range, then a protective action is required. The work is rejected. The work is repeated. Inspection is done again.

This protective action is separate from the control action just discussed. The aim of the control action is to get right on the target. The aim of the protective action is to make sure that the work is good enough to serve.

This sounds like go/no-go. Well, it is go/no-go, but only for the protective action.

Separating control from protection is an important conceptual step in learning to design robust systems—Six Sigma systems.

Show the rejection rate on a chart.

It stands to reason that good control performance will result in high success rates and low rejection rates.

Methods and Tools

26

Visualization

Charts provide management information and self-management information. Charts are a key tool for organizational performance.

CHECKLIST

☑ Charts say "This matter is important" and "Here's how we're doing."

☑ Feature performance charts in reports to management.

☑ Feature workplace postings of performance charts to reinforce objectives.

☑ Feature charts and other illustrations in communications to other interested parties.

VISUALIZATION

Illustrations tell the story compactly and save everybody's time. A picture is still worth a thousand words.

There are three target populations for charts and other visuals:

1. *Management.* Charts focus on key measures of performance and save management time.

2. *Self-management.* Charts in medical records highlight patient conditions and call the caregiver's attention to essential matters. Charts with control bands are even better because they call attention to any unexpected observations. The chart helps the caregiver do what the caregiver was going to do anyway, perhaps with a gentle reminder.

Charts posted in the workplace give work groups feedback on their performance. Charts, being impersonal, are less apt to get a negative reaction from employees than a supervisor conveying the same message. Maybe that's because the chart is not making any judgment, it is just stating the information.

3. *Nonspecialist audiences, including the public.* A chart says two things: this parameter is so important that we bother to keep close track of it, and here's how we're doing.

TRACKING CHARTS

Tracking charts plot each observation, one after the other, so that the lateral direction represents time or sequence. The vertical direction represents value. Figure 26.1 is a simple tracking chart repeated from

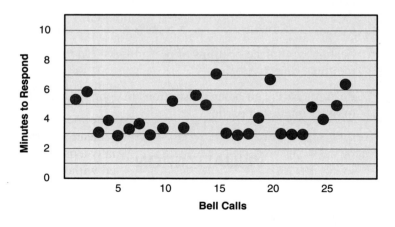

Figure 26.1 Patient service—time to respond to call bells.

a previous chapter. It shows performance for each of a sequence of about 25 events.

Many charts have control bands so that points falling outside the control band catch the eye and call out for further scrutiny. The control band may be imposed as a requirement, or the control band may just be a range in which, based on history, the points should be expected to fall most of the time.

Control bands based on history are commonly set at the historical mean plus and minus two standard deviations, with these standard deviations just being the standard deviation of the historical observations. If the control bands are set at plus and minus two standard deviations, then 95 percent of all observations should fall within the band. At plus and minus three standard deviations, 99.7 percent of all observations should fall within the band. Natural fluctuations would be expected to show one observation outside the 95 percent band about once a month if observations are taken daily, and about one observation outside the 99.7 percent band in a year. So, if points are showing up outside the control bands more often than that, something's going on that needs attention.

These control bands are based on the normal distribution, the familiar bell curve. The normal distribution is 'normal' because the sum of observations taken from distributions of any kind, or from any mix of distributions of any kind, is always normally distributed. That's the central limit theorem,[1] and it's handy because most things being observed are the result of several upstream or internal things going on.

If the chart is tracking observations that either happen or don't happen, such as the number of walk-in patients or the number of beds occupied, then a better way of doing the limits is to calculate the control limits by applying the Poisson distribution. The complication is that the standard deviation depends on the mean value in the Poisson distribution, so an estimate of the mean is required before the bands can be calculated. That's not usually a problem, and in the worst case, the tracking chart can be started without the control bands, and then the control bands can be added later.

---

1. See Keywords in Appendix A, page 205.

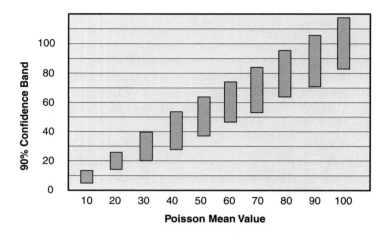

Figure 26.2   Poisson 90 percent bands.

Figure 26.2 shows the control bands corresponding to 90 percent coverage for a range of Poisson mean values. If values are plotted once a day, then about three observations per month can be expected to fall outside this 90 percent band. Calculating the control band limits for the Poisson distribution require only simple spreadsheet calculations using built-in functions. See page 210.

COMPARISON CHARTS

Comparisons can be done by plotting the points in various colors or using various plotting symbols, so that the aggregate and specific data all blend together.

Sometimes it is helpful to do a bar chart to make side-by-side comparisons in an obvious way. For instance, if some doctors are turning in their dictations within 24 hours of discharge and some are not, and there are many doctors involved, as is commonly the case, then a bar chart posted in a conspicuous place might get some cooperation. It's more apt to work than nagging. Each doctor can be assigned a letter of the alphabet so that the doctor knows which column to look at, and since the bars are otherwise anonymous,

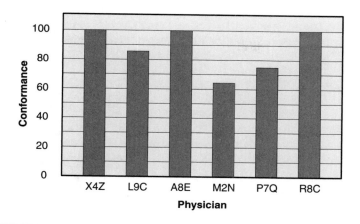

Figure 26.3 Use of preferred protocol.

there is no public embarrassment. Figure 26.3 is an example from a prior chapter.

The point here is to get some cooperation or self-management. It works surprisingly well.

VALUE-ADDED CHARTS

Value-added charts show, in a notional way, when some value is being added to the patient's treatment and when not. Figure 26.4 is an example.

A value-added chart for each patient will highlight holdups and give a target for expediting and resolving conflicts in priorities that are causing the holdups or delays.

A family of value-added charts for a population of patients receiving the same treatment will bring to light systematic problems and focus attention on resolution of same.

While value-added charts are helpful to any party interested in stage-by-stage service, they are particularly helpful to the case manager in the expediter role and to the service line manager interested in systematic improvement.

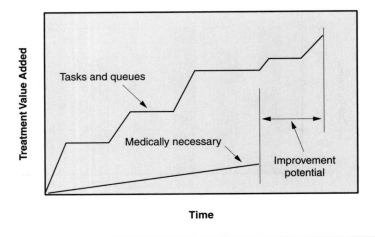

Figure 26.4   Value-added chart example.

TRIAL PROGRESS

For tracking successes and failures, case by case, and comparing to an expected performance level, a successive-events tracking chart is helpful. A specific application of this method was given in Chapter 3, page 11, for comparing local survival rates against national standards. Using this method is better than waiting until enough new data points are available to do textbook population comparisons. After all, this may well be life or death, so every case is vital in the true sense of the word.

In Figure 26.5, the band limits are calculated from confidence levels against false-positive and false-negative outcomes. Success is getting from the starting point, 1.000, down to the lower line. Failure is crossing the upper line. In the middle, judgment is suspended. Refer to Appendix D, page 223, for further information on the method.

The plotted points reveal more than would a table of numbers. Progress and setbacks are obvious, even to those who have no knowledge of the interworkings.

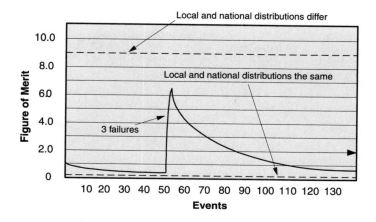

Figure 26.5   Sequential events tracking example.

UNCERTAINTY VERSUS THE ILLUSION OF CERTAINTY

Management deals with uncertainty all the time. The import of this chapter is to display information in such a way that information is conveyed without suppressing the uncertainty in what the next data point will show.

There are plenty of statistical analysis software packages that will fit lines to points, do multiple regressions, and calculate innumerable goodness-of-fit parameters to six or eight decimal places. Those are fine for statisticians working with mountains of data.

They are not helpful and often anti-helpful when applied by the nonspecialist to convey information to management because they create an illusion of certainty. "Significant at the 0.05 level" sounds good, but is it? It's saying that there is a five percent chance of being wrong, which might be okay for some matters and utterly unacceptable for others. Is being wrong once a month acceptable? One hour a day?

Except in research settings, there are rarely enough data to support multifactor regression analysis or other higher-order statistical analysis. Applying such methods to limited quantities of data can lead the user astray.

Better to stick to simple tracking charts, leaving the higher-order analysis to specialists and researchers.

27

DMAIC

Six Sigma process improvement goes through specific stages: define the objective, measure the baseline, analyze the baseline, implement trials, and control the results to be certain that improvements abide. These are commonly abbreviated as DMAIC.

CHECKLIST

☑ Understand the baseline.

☑ When you fix something, fix it all the way.

☑ Keep tracking to make sure the improvement abides.

☑ Keep the number of major projects down to a manageable few.

MANAGED CHANGE

While all process improvement methods have a step-by-step change management procedure, and while they all look pretty much the same, Six Sigma puts emphasis on a few fundamental points.

The Six Sigma steps are:

1. *D*efine the objective or performance requirement in numbers.

2. *M*easure the baseline, the preexisting process.

3. *A*nalysis and come to understand the baseline process.

4. *I*mplement change, using pilot programs first.

5. *C*ontrol the new process to make sure the improvements abide.

These points of particular emphasis with Six Sigma are explained in the following sections.

The four-step process called plan–do–check–act (PDCA), which is the grandfather of DMAIC, may be more familiar to the reader. The reason for adding another step will be discussed below.

Both DMAIC and PDCA use data to inform. They are not 'data-driven,' because no driving is going on. Informing, yes, driving, no. Decision making abides with the human beings.

UNDERSTAND THE BASELINE

Make a flowchart, page 177, so that interested parties can visualize what's going on in the sequential process. Worry in particular about the communications events.

The natural tendency is to see the shortcomings in the baseline and jump to conclusions about improvements.

But consider that smart people instituted the existing baseline, and they had reasons for everything they did. Without debating whether the present staff is even smarter, it is wise to start with the view that there was a reason for every step. Dig that reason out. Is that reason still valid? Is sufficient weight given to it in the proposed changes?

Using the three-plane model, page 185, examine existing policies that bear on the baseline. Are they still appropriate? Have external matters, such as regulations, changed the ground rules? Has there been a technology change? Capacity change?

Get data. If you don't have data on the existing condition, you won't be able to determine whether the 'improvement' improves anything or not.

Fix quantitative objectives and service levels. Ask whether the baseline could reasonably be expected to meet the objectives and service levels with more of something, such as diligence, training, or rework of the baseline, perhaps changing the sequence of events or assignment of responsibilities.

SOLVE IT

Foreswear incrementalism.

Every change is a bother. Find a solution that solves the whole issue once and for all, a solution that makes the objective and service level easy to meet.

Don't fiddle around with partial solutions. Don't mess with Mr. In-Between (page xxi).

If the improvement isn't worth the cost, then this is not a serious topic and is not worthy of management attention.

GET A GOOD PITCH TO HIT[1]

Management can only cope with a few changes at once if their impact crosses departmental lines, which almost all changes do.

Therefore, do a ranking of projects, and select the ones that make the most sense.

Positive features of a change are:

- Early benefit in resource utilization

- Conspicuous improvement as seen by the customers

- Competitive advantage

---

1. Ted Williams said that's the best batting advice he ever got. He got it from Rodgers Hornsby.

COST REDUCTION, LOWER PRIORITY

It is often said that junior management worries about cost reduction and senior management worries about the balance sheet.

Resource utilization shows up on the balance sheet.

This book focuses on resource utilization because improving resource utilization is a bigger lever on financial condition than is cost reduction. We are not opposed to cost reduction, and we believe that cost reduction is everybody's everyday job.

If Six Sigma methods are used locally to reduce costs, that's fine. Such projects, though, are probably not the ones that are going to be key to senior management.

WHAT'S DIFFERENT ABOUT DMAIC

Other than having an extra letter in its name, what is the underlying difference between DMAIC as espoused by Six Sigma and plan–do–check–act (PDCA) as practiced by the very best people for six or seven decades? There are two.

First, there is a new emphasis on understanding the baseline, the prior condition, including measurements. Quantify. Consider. Think about why things are the way they are, what can be learned from experience, and what workers actually do (which might be quite different from what the procedure sheet says to do). With manual operations, get input from the people doing the work. Get data. Collect anecdotes. Be prepared to measure the results of any change against the baseline.

Second, DMAIC emphasizes long-term tracking of results. Lots of changes are favorable in the short run, particularly if they are being implemented by the proponents of the change. When that ownership/enthusiasm wears off, the new results still need to be maintained, or else the whole thing was feckless. The only way to know is to track.

Plan–do–check–act is often shown as a spiral, the meaning being that as soon as one change is complete, get started on the next one. While that's fine for an overall system, where an improvement project here is followed in time by an improvement project over there, spiraling needs to be done cautiously in any one locale. It takes time for people to get the hang of anything new. It takes time to work down into the happy bottom of the bathtub curve (page 102). It takes time just to get the word out to other shifts. Better to make sure each change is big enough to bother with and to make fewer discrete changes over time in any locale.

Some process improvement systems encourage experimentation in small increments, trying things to see what happens, figuring that better outcomes will be found by this sort of intuitive hunting. That may be okay for aluminum rolling mill controls, but it doesn't have much place in healthcare. Six Sigma does not encourage this. Rather, Six Sigma encourages carefully considered changes with each done on a controlled pilot basis. *La prudence, toujours la prudence.*[2]

---

2. Borrowing from Frederick the Great and standing him on his head.

28
Flowcharts

Flowcharts visualize how things work in sequence. They are the starting point for understanding existing operations.

CHECKLIST

- ☑ Follow the flow of material things.
- ☑ Follow the creation of the medical record.
- ☑ Follow the information flow.

THE BASIC IDEA

Figure 28.1 shows a typical flowchart.

In this chart, seven tasks are identified. They show that work proceeds in order, and that task C, for example, relies on the results of tasks A and B.

Task D produces two outputs, one going to task E and one going to task F.

There are two eventual outputs, one downstream of task E and one downstream of task G.

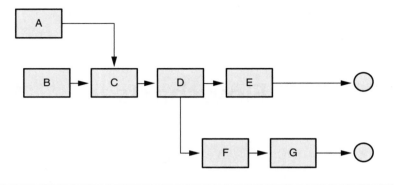

Figure 28.1   A typical flowchart.

Things flow from left to right. That's not a necessity, but it's generally easier to understand if that is so.

Flowcharts help people understand what's going on. That applies to people who are active within the process, because not everyone knows everything. People are often surprised to find out what's being done with their outputs, for example.

When healthcare flowcharts are made, there are questions to be asked, and answered for each box on the chart:

1. Who does this task?

2. Why is this task being done?

3. What inputs are required?

4. Who authorizes this task to begin?

5. Who decides when the task is completed?

6. Who verifies that the task is completed?

7. Who declares the task completed?

8. What are the outputs?

9. Who uses each output?

10. What evidence is generated?

11. What record is created?

12. Who is responsible for the record?

There are almost always some branches in a flowchart to cover options and conditional flows. Charts with such branches and decision points shown are often called *logic diagrams*. There is no material difference between a flowchart and a logic diagram.

There are quite often different shapes used for tasks, reports, decisions, and so on. These may be circles, triangles, diamonds, and other figures. While there are standards for these symbols in various industries, it is always a good idea to check on the meanings when looking at a new flowchart.

IMPROVING A PROCESS

Once the flowchart is drawn, it is appropriate to ask if the process can be improved. Improving the process almost always means shortening the time required to complete the process.

There are incentives to:

• Do more tasks in parallel.

• Combine tasks.

• Subdivide tasks.

• Change the sequence of tasks.

• Delete tasks.

The strongest urge is to delete tasks because that task hinders other matters. However, it needs always to be borne in mind that somebody who knew at the time what they were doing put this task in there for some reason. The reason may well have been lost in antiquity, but before any task is removed, careful thought needs to be given as to why it was put there in the first place. It might well have been valid, and the need may abide. Perhaps that need can be dealt with in a better way, but the only safe starting point is to assume that every task is there for some good reason.

INFORMATION FLOW

With manual tasks, which includes much of healthcare, it is vital that the information flow be well identified and well understood. Failures are much more apt to arise in communications than in some machine or in some oft-practiced task.

FAILURE MODES AND EFFECTS

Once the flowchart is in hand, and before any improvements are urged, it is helpful to consider each task and each transfer between tasks to see what might go wrong. What are the failure modes? What is the consequence of each potential failure?

Common sense can then rank these on a combined basis of seriousness of the consequences and likelihood of the failure. The ranked list is usually called a *critical items list.*

When changes in the flowchart are considered, it doesn't hurt to recheck the critical items list and the failure modes and effects. Improving A while inadvertently worsening B is not unknown.

It almost always works best to start at the right end of the flowchart and march to the left when doing this kind of analysis so that the number of extraneous possibilities doesn't get out of hand.

TRUST

Failure modes and effects analysis doesn't consider everything in the world, it considers things that are not entirely trustworthy. Trustworthy things are eliminated from consideration. What is trustworthy? A diagnosis confirmed by a second qualified practitioner. A kit of supplies from an established provider. Upstream work confirmed by inspection. An instrument recently calibrated.

Failure modes and effects analysis can be done from this perspective, and it is interesting to do so. Start with the things that merit trust, and narrow down the field to those things that do not merit trust. Since trust is necessarily a judgment call, it is illuminating to say, for each item, "I trust XYZ because . . . ."

IRREVERSIBILITY

Special attention needs to be paid to tasks that are irreversible. Make sure that any such tasks are well prepared before launching and that a time buffer is put in place just upstream so that people can take stock before launching.

COMBINING AND SUBDIVIDING TASKS

Combined tasks can often be done more readily. The trick is to make sure that no information is suppressed in the combining and that irreversible tasks are not inadvertently created or aggravated.

Tasks are subdivided for two reasons. One is to create intermediate inspection points so that the likelihood of success increases. The other is to create two different subtasks to serve two distinct output purposes. Using two stones to hit two birds is a Six Sigma design principle. See page 126.

One example was recently published in the *Wall Street Journal* (Wysocki 2004). In this case, a hospital wanted a medical technician to telephone each discharged patient to do a follow-up interview three days after discharge. That seems like a good idea. The technician was sent each medical record upon discharge so that the technician would know whom to telephone on the third day. Well, that meant that the record was being held for three days, which lengthened the billing and collection cycle by three days. Not good. So the task was subdivided so that the record went to the coding department and a small notice form was sent to the technician. Two birds. Two stones.

29

Chains of Events

In analyzing how things come to happen, it is necessary to consider the three distinct chains of events, which give rise to the material cause, the proximate cause, and the efficient cause.

CHECKLIST

☑ Find the chain of the underlying condition.

☑ Find the chain of the action that triggered the event.

☑ Find the chain that led the event-initiating person to be there and do that.

ARISTOTLE SAID . . .

Every event has three causes: the material cause, the proximate cause, and the efficient cause. By *efficient cause* he meant the person who triggered the whole thing (Aristotle 1952, 259 et. seq.).

Consider the straw that broke the camel's back. The material cause was the heavy load already on the camel. The proximate cause was that last straw. The efficient cause was the camel driver who put that last straw on the camel. Take away any one of these, and the camel's back survives another day.

Consider the Great Chicago Fire (CHS 1996). The material cause was the flammable structures of the barn and the city. The proximate cause was the lantern. The efficient cause was Mrs. O'Leary's cow. Or so the story goes. Take away any one of these, and that fire does not start that day in that location.

So, make three chains of events. One for the material cause. One for the proximate cause. One for the efficient cause.

CORRECTIVE ACTION

It is only necessary to break one of the chains and keep it broken.

It doesn't hurt to break two or all three, and indeed this would provide a defense in depth.

Having the three chains in mind clarifies thinking when corrective actions are proposed.

GENERALIZE

It is usually easy enough to trace the chains of events and identify things that fix the specific case.

The difficulty comes in trying to generalize, to find that management policy that takes care of this particular case and extends it in a useful way to preclude other cases from happening too. Easy to say, but how to do? For this, refer to the next chapter.

30
Planes of Resolution

Management benefits from viewing things on three planes: the mechanisms, the conditions, and the policies. This third plane is where management action is felt.

CHECKLIST

☑ Fill the mechanisms plane using chains of events and other such descriptors.

☑ Fill the conditions plane by identifying resources and operating conditions.

☑ Fill the policies plane with the policies, regulations, and other administrative actions that management can act upon.

THE MODEL

This model for analyzing events, planes of resolution, has been developed by the Federal Aviation Administration, the people who study every airplane crash in fine detail (Leveson 1995; Barry 2002, 48). See Figure 30.1. There are very few plane crashes, thankfully. There are not enough plane crashes to support statistical analysis,

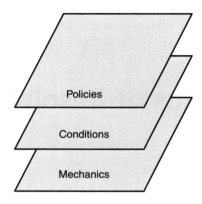

Figure 30.1 Planes of resolution.

the way car crashes are analyzed. Since there are few specimens to examine, much has to be learned from each one.

This is a good model for healthcare. Much has to be learned from every single negative experience.

The first plane, mechanisms, is straightforward. Trace the chains of events and the sequence of events. Find comparable parallels, if possible, where the outcome was favorable so that essential differences can be spotted.

The second plane, conditions, also is straightforward. What capital equipment was available? Were the workers qualified? What was the weather? What else was going on that distracted attention? What signs were missed? What regulations applied?

The third plane, policies, are things under management control. What was the staffing policy? What was the training policy? What was the capacity policy?

MANAGEMENT APPLICATION

To the extent that the cause of a difficulty was strictly mechanical or a failure of a trained person to follow the training, then corrective measures can be taken at lower levels, and reoccurrence is unlikely.

To the extent, however, that reoccurrence cannot be ruled out, then middle and senior management should look carefully at the third plane, policies. Which policy needs further attention? What would be the trade-offs if a policy change were to be made? How can a policy change be evaluated on a trial basis of some sort? What can be learned from others that might be helpful?

Indeed, does management need to seek to influence outside agencies, such as regulators, to attain the necessary improvement by changing the conditions that appear on the second plane?

Let's use this model to evaluate the Great Chicago Fire of 1871. The story in brief: There were barns in the city because people needed milk and transportation. Chicago had two fires on a typical day and had plenty of fire telegraphs (call boxes) and pumpers to handle two fires. Then one day, a day like all days, one fire took hold and overwhelmed the firefighting systems. Consider what city management had on its plate. It could not change the weather, it could not outlaw barns, it could not outlaw lanterns. Okay, so what could it do? Well, it could mandate that wide avenues be built every quarter of a mile to act as a fire break. It could mandate that every barn have a bucket of sand. It could . . . . What would you suggest? It was 1871 remember, so no laser beams, if you please.

31
Trials

Changes are to be tried before they are implemented generally.

CHECKLIST

☑ Have the baseline well quantified.

☑ Set high goals.

☑ Quantify trial results.

☑ Provide off-ramps, just in case.

☑ Have a fallback position, because the trial is just a trial.

POTENTIAL PROBLEM ANALYSIS

As soon as a change is proposed for trial, management should institute a potential problem analysis by getting as many negative thinkers as possible in the room and ask them to list all the things that might go wrong. Positive thinkers don't contribute much at this stage.

With the potential problems identified, the trial should be adapted, if possible, to overcome the potential problems. While this takes some judgment, it is a necessary part of the dynamic.

The as-modified proposal can then be reevaluated to see if it is still worth taking to trial. If not, it's time to consider other candidates.

Potential problem analysis should include failure modes and effects analysis, page 133, but should go further. Failure modes and effects analysis tends to be rather mechanical. Potential problem analysis should go on to conjure up other things, such as employee reaction, conflicts with other changes going on elsewhere, and known future changes in regulations. Think wide, as well as negatively.

TRIAL MANAGEMENT

Management can only deal with a small number of multidepartment projects at once, so a ranking of candidates is necessary.

For those selected, a project manager is required along with necessary support personnel. A steering group of departmental middle managers can be helpful.

Each trial should have specific, quantitative objectives and service levels with tracking plans and charts in hand.

Every trial is necessarily a test of the hypothesis that the proposed system is better than the baseline. Since quantitative baseline information is in hand, there are analytic methods available to confirm/refute that the hypothesis[1] is supportable. One interesting way is described in Appendix F, page 235, which provides for evaluation of success/failure for each sequential application of the trial.

TRIAL DISCIPLINE

Healthcare is procedure-oriented. Everything to be done is written down, every person to be doing the thing is trained ahead of time.

And yet it is in the nature of trials that surprises will happen. Participants will discover changes that should be made. Awkward tasks will become obvious. Things will jump out.

---

1. The hypothesis is always stated the other way around, making the null hypothesis that there is no change. The reason for this is that nobody has found a way to do the arithmetic except for null hypotheses.

It is sorely tempting to make changes on the fly. If the trial is being done in a sandbox, it might be for the best to make such changes on the fly. In non-sandbox cases, that simply cannot be done. Take notes and make recommendations, but don't make changes on the fly.

OFF-RAMPS

Part of the trial design is to identify off-ramps, which are places in the trial where the trial will be stopped. The signals for the off-ramps need to be identified as part of the trial plan.

It is better to take an off-ramp and start over again than to adjust the trial on the fly.

REVERSIBILITY

Make sure that the trial is just a trial and that the prior situation is not destroyed while the trial is going on. The trial may fail. A fallback position needs to be maintained.

EVALUATION

Did the trial show that the issue was dealt with in a final and clear way? The objective should be to overcome the difficulty completely, not to make improvements at the margin. That's because change is a burden on management, and there is only so much management capacity. Find improvements that are worth management's time and energy.

32

Sustained Improvement

Trials often succeed just because they are being done by enthusiasts. To verify that the gains are sustainable requires persistent, long-term tracking.

CHECKLIST

☑ Plan for a long period of sustained evaluation.

☑ Track against objective criteria.

☑ Plan off-ramps, just in case.

ENTHUSIASM VERSUS STRUCTURAL IMPROVEMENT

The trial will be conducted by enthusiasts. The general application will be carried out by some enthusiasts plus a lot of competent but disinterested persons. The test of sustainability is whether only enthusiasts can get the positive results.

This can be addressed before general implementation by having a second trial period with other people assigned, in some cases. Still, there will be some uncertainty about sustained improvement until it is demonstrated on its own.

OBJECTIVE CRITERIA

When the change is implemented, track against objective and aggressive criteria. The test isn't whether the new system is better than the old one, the test is whether the new system solves the issue once and for all.

OFF-RAMPS

Prepare signals and actions to stop the general implementation if bad news happens. This preparation will likely include tracking additional parameters and collecting anecdotal views from participants and others.

POINT OF NO RETURN

If the *trial* fails, the organization simply reverts to the prior condition.

If the *general application* fails, can the organization reverse course and re-implement the prior condition? How long can management support keeping the reversibility option open?

In long-distance flying, this is known as the point of no return. At that point, the plane is better off going on to the destination than returning to the starting point.

The same applies to any change. There is a point when management necessarily decides to go ahead or to go back. If ahead, then management clears away the support systems for the old operation and commits to the new.

This is a major decision. It should be made at the appropriate senior level and on the basis of lots of information.

Senior Management To-Do

33

Specific Management Actions

Organizations respond to what the senior management conveys by thought, word, and deed. Ask for high achievement, you may well get it. Others have.

CHECKLIST

☑ Set high targets.

☑ Get board, chief medical officer (CMO), and chief nursing officer (CNO) support.

☑ Select patient-oriented objectives.

☑ Set measures for progress.

☑ Communicate.

THE ROLE OF SENIOR MANAGEMENT

Nothing much is going to happen in any organization that is opposed by senior management, and nothing much is going to happen that is simply ignored by senior management.

Senior management sets the tone.

That's good. That's where the responsibility should rest.

Experience in the relatively short history of Six Sigma is that when top management embraces Six Sigma, good things happen quickly, and favorable results are sustained. The best-known case is that of Jack Welch, who was CEO of GE, one of the biggest and most complex companies in the world. Welch, who holds a PhD in chemical engineering and who had a wide range of management responsibilities in his GE career, learned of Six Sigma from one of his board members. Seeing the positive potential, Welch issued an order saying that all GE persons applying for any management position would henceforth have at least Green Belt[1] certification in Six Sigma.

The organization turned to. Here was a communication that people understood. Welch had matched word and deed. Welch, now retired, continues to remark that Six Sigma was one of the keys to GE's success during his remarkable tenure.

It is to be noted that GE was already one of the best managed companies in the world with highly sophisticated quality methods. Even so, Welch thought they could do better, and the record shows that they did do better by applying Six Sigma to all aspects of their businesses, and not just to factory work. GE is a huge financial services company, and the financial services unit quickly found benefit in applying Six Sigma.

Maybe they would have found those same benefits anyway no matter what the program in vogue happened to be, and maybe not. Welch believes that Six Sigma made a step change in GE's performance. Who's to say he's wrong?

Welch set the tone. Welch declared policy. Welch caused the promotion/reward system to be adapted to support the policy. Welch looked to his business unit managers to follow through.

GE is a positive example of Six Sigma. There are other wonderful examples:

- Mount Carmel Hospitals, Columbus, Ohio, which is part of the Trinity group. www.mchs.com

- Heritage Valley Healthcare System, Beaver and Sewickley, Pennsylvania. www.hvhs.org

---

1. See page 3 for information on Six Sigma 'belts.'

- Boca Raton Community Hospital, Boca Raton, Florida. www.brch.com

This section of the book covers, in brief, those matters any senior management has to address with any new strategic policy. These are the classic business text topics: setting the objective, planning, organizing, staffing, directing, evaluating, coordinating, and controlling. They are gathered here in one place as lists for the convenience of the reader.

They are, we believe, a coherent set. Taken together, they provide the highest likelihood of success. Even taken piecemeal, each makes a positive contribution.

OBJECTIVES

- Conform the organization's objectives to the patient's objectives.

- Aim for substantial and verifiable improvement in important matters clearly related to patient safety, patient service, and patient care.

PLANNING

- Select a planning horizon over a number of quarters, with quarterly reviews.

- Provide time for learning at senior levels.

- Get chief medical officer, chief nursing officer, and board agreement.

- Pick early actions that cost little or nothing and that are likely to improve resource utilization, including evidence-based medicine, clinical pathways, and patient pathways as prescribed in earlier chapters.

- Build on success.

ORGANIZING

- Assign service line managers to patient populations.
- Assign profit responsibility to service line managers.
- Put the chief nursing officer on the same rank as the chief medical officer.

STAFFING

- Conform to Magnet Nursing standards.
- Ensure that the workplace is blame-free.
- Provide ample training and retraining in all aspects of healthcare.
- Provide specific training in Six Sigma matters so that the benefits will be internalized and institutionalized, rather than relying on outside consultants.

DIRECTING

- Urge the medical staff to select evidence-based protocols for each medical condition.
- Urge the medical staff and nursing staff to establish clinical and patient pathways with tracking charts and control bands for patient parameters.
- Select a patient protection topic for deep study and possible improvement.
- Select an operations topic with resource implications.
- Select a patient service topic based on in-hand patient satisfaction surveys.

EVALUATING

- Require tracking charts to be included in all reports to senior management.

- Require third-party evaluations of all claims of improvement in resource utilization or patient care. These may be in-house evaluations, provided the evaluators are distinct from enthusiasts.

COORDINATING

- Select only a few projects crossing departmental lines to minimize the coordination burden.

- Coordinate between Six Sigma projects and other mandatory projects.

CONTROLLING

- Track resource utilization improvements.

Appendices

Appendix A
Specialized Vocabulary

A review of vocabulary and a set of useful spreadsheet functions.

KEYWORDS

Here are some words and definitions.

mean value—To determine, add up all the observations and divide by the number of observations.

average value—This is the same as the mean value.

variance—To determine, square and add up the differences between each observed value and the mean value. Divide by the number of observations.

standard deviation—This is the square root of the variance. The lowercase Greek letter *sigma* (σ) is often used for standard deviation. Consequently, σ^2 is used for the variance.

distribution—This is the probability of each possible occurrence of the variable. By convention, the sum of all probabilities is unity; the distribution is scaled, or normalized, so that the total probability is unity. Common distributions are the normal distribution, the uniform distribution, the binominal distribution, and the Poisson distribution. There are many others.

cumulative distribution—This is the probability that the next sample will be to the left of the selected value of the variable. This is found by adding up all the probabilities to the left.

median value—This is the value of the variable for which the cumulative distribution is equal to 50 percent. The probability of the next observation falling to the left is 50 percent, to the right is 50 percent. The *median* value and the *mean* value will be the same if the distribution is symmetric, otherwise not.

central limit theorem—Make observations from several distributions. Add them up. The sum will have the normal distribution. Note that the several distributions can be of any kind or any mix of kinds of distributions. (Each must have a finite standard deviation, but that's a trivial requirement in real life.) Since most things that are observed in real-life situations are the result of several things happening over a series of steps, most observed happenings have the normal distribution.

law of large numbers—Make observations from any distribution. Calculate the mean of the observations. The likelihood increases with observation count that the mean value of the underlying (and unknown) distribution is close to the mean of the observations. This is sometimes called the *strong law of large numbers.* There is also a *weak law of large numbers* that says the standard deviation of the underlying distribution is approximated by the standard deviation of the observations, but the quality of this estimate increases only with the square root of the number of observations, so this is weaker than the strong relationship for estimating the mean value.

histogram—A histogram is a plot of observation counts against the value of the variable. For continuous variables, divide the range into convenient intervals. The histogram will, for a reasonable number of samples, reveal the general shape of the underlying distribution being sampled.

THE NORMAL DISTRIBUTION

The shape of the distribution curve in Figure A.1 is the familiar bell-shaped curve, which is called the *normal distribution* and sometimes

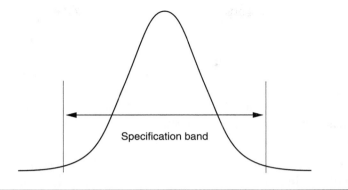

Figure A.1   Normal distribution with specification band.

the *Gaussian distribution.* This is the most common distribution because the result of any process involving multiple steps tends to look like this. This tendency is called the *central limit theorem.*

The variable can in theory take on all values from minus infinity to plus infinity; however, the probability of the variable taking on extreme values is extremely tiny. Ninety-five percent of the area under the curve is within two standard deviations of the mean value.

The normal curve has two parameters: its mean value and its standard deviation. These are independent of one another.

Given the mean and the standard deviation, the distribution itself can be determined by looking up values in a printed table or by using spreadsheet functions. More often, the matter of interest is determining the fraction of the total area under the curve that falls between two points. For instance, what is the area between minus one standard deviation and plus one standard deviation? Or, what is the area to the right of plus 4.5 standard deviations? Since the total area under the curve is 100 percent by definition, these calculated areas correspond to the probability that the next observation will fall into that particular range. These areas are computed readily by spreadsheet functions. Some are discussed here.

• *Control band* or *specification band.* Figure A.1 shows a specification band. By inspection, a large fraction of samples drawn from this distribution will fall within this band. To monitor any such process, it is helpful to establish a band and observe what fraction, over time, of the samples fall within the band and what fraction fall outside the band. Some judgment is required in setting the width of the band. The band should be set so that a point falling outside the band is sufficiently unlikely that attention is warranted. For instance, if the band is set wide enough to cover 99 percent of expected occurrences, then a point falling outside the band may just be a random occurrence or it may be a message that the process has changed somehow and that the process needs to be verified. Attention, at least to verify the process, is warranted.

• *Control chart* and *tracking chart*. Both charts present data point by point, almost always in historical order, left to right. Both charts have bands marked to show where the points are expected to fall so that exceptional points catch the eye. The band for a tracking chart need not have any formula basis and may just show expected direction of movement for future data points. A control chart has control bands (see Figure A.1) calculated formally from prior data or from an engineering model of the process with the band width set at plus and minus three standard deviations so that all but one percent of data points can be expected to fall within the band in the normal course of events. That is to say, a point falling outside this band calls for attention but not necessarily for action. Control charts often have an additional band at plus and minus four standard deviations or some other such number at which point action is to be taken. Points fall outside these bands so infrequently that there is a presumption of process upset calling for prompt action. Control charts are generated for individual data points, for the average value of a batch of points, and for the variance within a batch of values. Control charts and tracking charts are most commonly used to inform operators and other interested parties while things are going on, although they can be of some use later on to figure out when something subtle happened.

OTHER DISTRIBUTIONS OF INTEREST

Some things are distributed *uniformly*. Look at your watch and observe the second hand. That observation will be uniformly distributed from zero to 60. The uniform distribution has two parameters, the minimum and maximum values. Note, however, that it does not have tails. The only way to deal with parameters that are uniformly distributed is to make sure the target band is wide enough to tolerate everything between the minimum and the maximum. Or, work on the process to move the minimum or maximum or both.

Variables that can take on only one or the other of two values are distributed *binomially*. The *binomial distribution* has two parameters, the probability that the preferred value appears and the total population count. So, if 20 patients are scheduled and if experience shows that any one patient will show up with a probability of 90 percent, then the binomial distribution tells us the chance of having 16 or 17 or 18 or 19 or 20 patients showing up on a particular day. (It's nine percent, 19 percent, 29 percent, 27 percent, and 12 percent, respectively.) Or as a practical matter the question might be, what's the probability that 18 to 20 patients will show up? (It's 68 percent.)

The binomial distribution looks something like a bell-shaped curve, but it has a finite range running from zero to the total population. It has tails away from the mean value, but they do not run to infinity.

An interesting special case of the binomial distribution is the *Poisson* distribution. The Poisson distribution applies if only a few out of some very large population actually participate in some event. For instance, a savings bank with ten thousand depositors might find that about 20 show up during the Thursday lunch hour and 50 show up at Friday lunch hour. Banks, grocery stores, and emergency departments can make productive use of the Poisson distribution to forecast demand for service.

The Poisson distribution is unusual in that only one parameter is required, the mean value. So, if 40 is the average number of emergency room patients who turn up on Saturday nights with a full moon, then the Poisson distribution says that the likelihood of at least 35 showing up the next such Saturday evening is 76 percent, and the likelihood that more than 45 will show up is 19 percent.

The Poisson distribution is limited in range on the left because the variable can be no less than zero for the good reason that the number of passengers, say, cannot be negative. It is not limited on the right because an infinite number of passengers *might* show up; however, the distribution falls off rapidly to the right of the mean value, so the tail of the distribution on the right is small.

The Poisson distribution is discussed further in Appendix D on the *Erlang distributions.* See page 223. Erlang distributions deal with finite capacity systems faced with variable demand, which is what every healthcare facility is.

Failure patterns over time often exhibit a *bathtub* shape, high at the beginning, low in the middle, and then rising again later. Lots of electronic and mechanical systems show this behavior; so do people. See page 102.

SPREADSHEET FUNCTIONS

All modern spreadsheets have built-in functions that do elementary statistical operations. The function names here are for Microsoft Excel. Other spreadsheets may have slightly different names and arrangements of arguments.

- *Average (…).* This computes the average value of a set. The average = mean value.

- *Stdev (…).* This computes the standard deviation of a set.

- *Normdist (x, mean, standard deviation, cumulative flag).* This function returns the value of the normal distribution for variable = x, given the mean and standard deviation for the distribution. If the cumulative flag is set to TRUE, then the function returns the cumulative value, which is the area under the distribution curve to the left of variable = x and is also equal to the probability that the next sample will fall to the left of x.

- *Binomdist (x, population, probability, cumulative flag).* This returns the value of the binomial distribution for variable = x, given a total population and the probability parameter. The cumulative flag is either TRUE or FALSE.

- *Poisson (x, mean, cumulative flag).* Note that the Poisson distribution requires a mean value as a parameter, not a probability nor a population size.

- *Histogram.* Excel will plot a histogram for a set. See Excel Help for details.

- Excel will also do well-known statistical tests such as the *chi-square* test and the *Student-t* test. These go beyond our immediate needs but can be of interest, sometimes, in comparing observations from two distributions (usually, to find out if the two are the same or not). In real-life situations, these tests rarely tell the user any more than overlaid plots of the two sets of samples will reveal, so they will not be elaborated here.

- Excel will also fit straight lines to data points and even do multifactor fits (*regressions*). These should be used most judiciously in real-life situations because the number of observations available is rarely enough to provide highly confident fits to the data.

Appendix B
Six Sigma Arithmetic

A brief explanation of why 3.4 per million is associated with Six Sigma.

CHECKLIST

☑ Six Sigma allows for controllable and uncontrollable variability.

☑ Six Sigma allows for drift.

☑ Six Sigma principles apply to all manner of distributions; the familiar 3.4 per million applies to the normal distribution.

☑ It's not the number that counts. It's the aggressive goal and the matching discipline that count.

VARIABILITY

All processes have some variability. That variability includes two kinds: controllable variability and uncontrollable variability. Both exist at all times. Uncontrollable variability is inherent to the process as it exists. For example, patients respond differently to medication. Controllable variability is everything else and is subject to detection and corrective action.

DRIFT

In addition to instantaneous variability, many processes exhibit a drift over time. The whole distribution moves. This can be viewed as a drift in the mean value of the distribution. Since this happens, it is necessary to take it into consideration.

The drift may be periodic. For instance, work teams on different shifts may have different levels of success. Or the drift may be monotonic, due perhaps to aging of equipment being used.

TAILS OF THE DISTRIBUTION

Standard tables and spreadsheet functions provide the size of the tails of common distributions.

The tails are the portions outside the desired band. The size of the tail, expressed as a fraction, is the probability that the next event will fall outside the desired band.

Sometimes only the tail to the right is of interest, sometimes only the tail to the left, sometimes both.

Table B.1 shows tail sizes for ranges of interest for the normal distribution.

THE SIX SIGMA MAGIC NUMBER

Six Sigma is commonly associated with the number 3.4 per million. By inspection of Table B.1, 3.4 per million corresponds to one-sided tails at plus or minus 4.5 standard deviations. This measurement, 4.5, is not six. How does this work?

The logic is as follows:

1. Start with six standard deviations in mind.

2. Allow 1.5 standard deviations for drift of the mean.

Table B.1 Normal distribution tails.

Value, in standard deviations	Tail to left	Tail to right	Both tails
−1	15.9%		
+1		15.9%	
2 (−1 to +1)			31.7%
−1.5	6.7%		
+1.5		6.7%	
3 (−1.5 to +1.5)			13.4%
−2.25	1.2%		
+2.25		1.2%	
4.5 (−2.25 to + 2.25)			2.4%
−3	0.1%		
+3		0.1%	
6 (−3 to +3)			0.2%
−4.5	3.4E−6*		
+4.5		3.4E−6	
9 (−4.5 to +4.5)			6.8E−6

* E−6 means 10 to the negative sixth power. In this case, this gives 3.4 per million.

3. That leaves 4.5 standard deviations for instantaneous variability.

4. Consider one-sided tails only.

5. The table says 3.4 per million for one-sided tails at 4.5 standard deviations.

If the process follows some other distribution, such as the Erlang distribution, the same sort of table can be constructed and applied.

BUT WHY SIX AND NOT SOME OTHER NUMBER OF SIGMAS?

Classical industrial process control starts with the notion that one rejection out of a thousand is a well-run process. From Table B.1, that will be seen to correspond to one-sided tails at plus or minus three standard deviations. The implication is that the specification for the results of the process match up with that much deviation in the process, so that 99.9 percent of the product conforms to specification.

If the specification is tightened, more product will be rejected, at least until the process is improved and can meet the tighter specification.

Motorola decided to do better, to deliver products with such uniformity in conformance to specification that a much, much lower fraction fall outside of specification. While this might be expressed in various ways, Motorola decided to do it by doubling the traditional measure, three standard deviations, to six standard deviations.[1]

Call it marketing, giving the market twice the performance previously expected. Call it inspiration. It worked.

Getting there required rethinking all phases of production. That's the whole point. That's why Six Sigma management and the Six Sigma tool kit can be applied not only to the factory but to the office and even to healthcare.

The step improvement in performance required setting aggressive goals and following through with management and methods and tooling and training and culture to get there.

---

1. Personal communication, Ed Popovich, PhD Vice President Enterprise Excellence, Boca Raton Community Hospital, formerly an executive with Motorola.

Appendix C
The Experience Curve

The Experience Curve is a rule of thumb that says productive effort continues to fall as experience with production rises. This relationship can be expressed in a simple way, and it seems to apply to a wide range of human experience.

CHECKLIST

☑ Expect productive effort to fall with experience.

☑ Standardize to get the benefit.

PARETO PRINCIPLE

Many readers will be aware of the Pareto principle, which says that 20 percent of a population generate 80 percent of the activity. Vilfredo Pareto was an Italian economist who wondered in 1908 why 20 percent of landowners in Italy owned 80 percent of the land (Reh 2002). This eventually came to be seen as a very general rule of thumb that applies so widely that it should be assumed to apply if there is no direct information to the contrary. For instance, 20 percent of telephone users generate 80 percent of the calling traffic (Briley 1983, 151). Why this should be, no one seems to know. Yet, there it is.

EXPERIENCE CURVE

There is a similar rule of thumb, which has one parameter, and remarkably enough, the parameter value is generally found to be around 20 percent. Perhaps there is some hidden relationship with the Pareto principle, perhaps this is coincidence. This second rule of thumb is embodied in the Experience Curve.

The underlying notion of the Experience Curve is that production gets better with experience. That doesn't seem radical; one might expect production to get better with experience. What is perhaps surprising is that production keeps getting better and better forever. Can that be? Well, it seems to be so.

Production, or productive effort as it is sometimes stated, refers to any of the factors of production—land, labor, or capital. It takes less of these factors as experience with production grows. Production becomes more efficient, so per-unit inputs are converted more efficiently to outputs. Perhaps capital is substituted for labor, or conceivably labor is substituted for capital, and the result is a net improvement in productive effectiveness and efficiency.

Experience is the accumulated repetition of production. Experience is measured in total units produced over time.

The relationship given by the Experience Curve is this: productive effort goes down 20 percent with each doubling of experience. Figure C.1 shows this simple relationship as a straight line (on ratio scales!). As experience grows from one unit produced to 1024 units produced, productive effort goes down by a factor of 10.

That's a lot. Now, the rule says that productive effort will continue to go down 20 percent with each doubling of experience, so on this same scale, if productive effort is 10 units when unit #1024 is produced, it will be about eight units when unit #2048 is produced. And so on. Unit #1,000,000 will require only about one unit of productive effort.

What's more, this keeps going.

The Experience Curve is plotted against production count, not time. To see what the effect is over time, it is necessary to know the rate of production per year, say. If it happens that the rate of production doubles every year, then the productive effort will fall 20

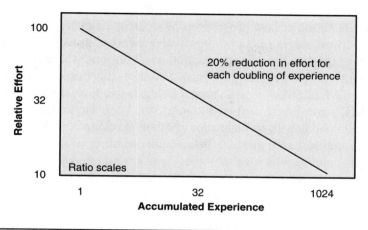

Figure C.1   Experience curve.

percent per year. If production goes up even faster, then productive effort will fall even faster, when plotted against a time scale.

Consider personal computers. Consider cell phones. Production rates have skyrocketed and unit costs of production have fallen like a rock. These all follow the Experience Curve, and they are conspicuous examples of what happens when the rate of productive increase is so quick as to make the results obvious.

Applied to mature products, the Experience Curve still applies, but the impact may be less obvious because the time scale expands. For instance, around 200,000,000 babies have been born in U.S. hospitals since at-home birthing went out of style 60 or so years ago. Mothers and babies, in those days, stayed in the hospital for a week or 10 days. Now it's one or two days. How long will it take to get the next 20 percent gain in productive effort related to maternity? At the present rate of births, which is around 4,000,000 per year, it will take 50 years to double the experience with this particular sort of production. Does it seem unreasonable that better methods, better equipment, better training, better technology will improve things by 20% over 50 years? Even productive methods that have been around very, very long times are still candidates for gains in efficiency.

(Gestation itself still takes 10 moons. Some things abide.)

Let's look at how progress in productive efficiency is made. In the earliest stages, reducing productive effort is mostly a matter of getting used to the new production, figuring out where inputs are being wasted, and getting the hang of things. Later on, better tooling is applied, not least because production gets to a high enough level to justify some investment in tooling. Still later, larger facilities are brought online with specialization of labor and equipment. Meanwhile, study and research produce better understanding of the underlying process and ancillary technologies such as computers and communications are brought to bear. This is almost never the result of one person or one group, it is the result of many persons doing their own part for their own reasons.

Take tooling. Tooling specialists develop new and specialized tooling if and when they are motivated to do so. Such specialists can pick the things they want to bother with, and they are most apt to pick a topic that will have the widest application, if only to make the maximum return on their own efforts.

This becomes self-reinforcing. More and more people, for their own reasons, work on the most popular targets, which accelerates the learning for the benefit of all participants. This is Adam Smith's 'invisible hand' at work (Smith 1776).

The impact of this for healthcare is that most interested parties will apply themselves for their own reasons to the most popular medical topics and tend to reinforce the most popular medical protocols. These days, those are the evidence-based medicine protocols. Less effort goes into improving nonstandard protocols, which tend to fall behind.

From time to time, research provides a step change in the standard method. These step improvements keep the Experience Curve going, and plotted on the appropriate scale, often fall on that same straight line.

Some productive processes continue in about the same way for centuries, such as getting milk from cows. Better nutrition, better sanitation, better machinery, better breeding—all keep the productive effort going in the same favorable direction. Some products have a short market life, such as eight-track tapes, and barely reach maturity. Medical protocols tend to be somewhere in between.

PERSISTENCE

The Experience Curve rewards persistence. Jumping around among production methods doesn't accumulate experience and therefore doesn't drive down productive effort requirements.

Standardize, persist, and incorporate better tooling, better training, and better facilities as they become available to reinforce the standard protocols and methods.

Appendix D
The Erlang Distributions

The Erlang distributions provide statistical models for systems with discrete, finite capacities. Originally developed for telephony, they apply equally well to healthcare capacity analysis with and without queuing.

CHECKLIST

☑ Erlang B for modeling systems with no queuing; excess demand goes elsewhere. Spreadsheet calculations are available.

☑ Erlang C for modeling systems with queuing, excess demand goes into the queue. Online calculations are available for free.

TRAFFIC ENGINEERING

Traffic engineering is the term applied in the telephone world to the study of finite capacities subjected to statistically-varying demand. Today, incremental capacity is cheap, but not long ago, adding one long distance circuit between two cities meant adding another wire all the way at great expense. So, incremental capacity represented a high fixed cost and was not undertaken lightly. The same applies to healthcare today. Adding one doctor to an emergency department is a high cost.

Telephony was one of the first industries to hire mathematicians to study practical problems. Bell Labs became famous worldwide for this, and other telephone companies made their own contributions. One such was the Copenhagen Telephone Company, which, in 1908, hired Agner Krarup Erlang, who set about thinking about how to analyze discrete-capacity systems.

Erlang started by thinking about the traffic. The question posed by Erlang to himself was: what are the chances that all circuits (or telephone operators or . . .) will be busy when the next customer tries to place a call? Then he went further to figure out how to size capacity to provide given levels of service in two cases: one, the rejected caller goes away; the other, the rejected caller waits in queue for service. (He also considered the case that the rejected caller tries again immediately, which doesn't appear to match up with most aspects of medical care, although it does apply to patients calling in from home to a doctor's office and who refuse to talk to an answering machine.)

First, Erlang convinced himself, mathematically, that so long as the total population out there that *might* seek service at any moment is very large, but the probability is small, and so long as the likelihood of a service being completed in the next short time interval is independent of the length of that service, then the quantity of traffic has the Poisson distribution. Erlang did not presume that the Poisson distribution would apply, he figured out the math for the traffic and observed that the formulas are the same as the Poisson formulas.

A peculiarity of the Poisson distribution is that the probability value is not known. Only the average occurrence is known, or observed. So for telephone calling, it is not a question of what the probability is that any one caller out of some large population is going to make a call during the time period of interest, only the average number of calls × the average duration of the call matters. This can be observed and determined by observation for like time periods.

The total traffic during the period of interest is what counts. For medical care, that's the total number of contact hours (doctors seeing patients) during the hours of interest. This is expressed in doctor-hours per period-of-interest hours. The ratio has the units of doctors-worth. The more general unit for traffic level is the *erlang,* which is the unit assigned by the International Organization for Standardization (ISO).

THE POISSON DISTRIBUTION

Start with events that either happen or do not happen. A patient comes in or that patient does not come in. It's one or the other. It's binomial (taking on only one or the other of two values). Flip a coin 17 times, using a fairly balanced coin having a probability of coming up heads of 50.0 percent. Repeat this several times. How often will exactly 12 tosses give heads and the other five give tails? The probability of seeing 12 heads and five tails given a population of 17 coins and a probability of success equal to 50 percent is given by the binomial distribution. The answer happens to be 4.7 percent. That is to say, if the trial of 17 flips is repeated 20 times, it is reasonable to expect that one of those sets will show exactly 12 heads. The other 19 trials will probably show some other number of heads. If this trial of 17 flips is repeated 200 times or 2000 times, one can be even more confident that there will be 12 heads 4.7 percent of the time.

The binomial distribution is well known and available in any computer spreadsheet.

The binominal distribution has two parameters: the probability value (the likelihood of success on the next trial) and the population size. The probability value is some number between zero and unity. The variance of the binomial distribution depends on the mean value and is given by (probability of success) × (1 − probability of success). The variance will be observed to be a maximum when the probability is near 50 percent and small when the probability is near zero or near unity. The standard deviation is the square root of the variance, by definition.

Sometimes, the total population is quite large and the fraction participating is quite small. For instance, a bank may have 10,000 depositors, only 23 of whom show up at the bank's teller windows during the Tuesday lunch hour. It would be convenient to have a distribution model that was more directly applicable to this situation than the binomial distribution.

The Poisson model fills this bill.

The Poisson model has only one parameter, which is the expected number of successes. The Poisson model assumes that the population is very large.

That's all that's required to produce the Poisson model. It has a formula, which is:

$$p(n; \mu) = \mu^n e^{-\mu} / n!$$

where n is the number of successes and μ is the average number of successes. All values for n are allowed, from zero to infinity, although the probability falls away very quickly for values of n any distance from the mean. The average need not be an integer; 13.79 is a perfectly good value for μ.

The variance of the Poisson distribution depends on the mean value and in fact is equal to the mean. The standard deviation is the square root of the variance.

The Poisson distribution looks like a bell curve if the mean value is much larger than about 10. If the mean value is small, then the distribution seems distorted and looks like it is squeezed in between zero and the mean, which of course it is.

The variable n can take on the value zero, because it is possible that the number of successes is zero. It may not be likely, but it is possible, and the distribution needs to cover all possibilities.

The sum of probabilities over all values of n from zero to infinity is exactly 100 percent. That's always the case for a probability distribution.

THE ERLANG B DISTRIBUTION

Erlang's question, posed to himself, was: what's the likelihood that every unit of capacity is already taken? He decided that the likelihood was equal to the value of the Poisson distribution for that number of units.

Suppose the capacity is c units and the mean is μ, the mean being known from prior experience. Then the likelihood of exactly c units being occupied at any one instant in time is the Poisson formula above with $n = c$.

Now suppose that all higher levels of traffic are ignored, those being refused service or transferred elsewhere for service. No queue, just service or not. With the tail chopped off, the sum of all probabilities is no longer unity as required by a probability distribution, so renormalization is required. The renormalization is done by adding up the probabilities of the allowed states, zero up to c, and using that as a scaling factor. This gives the Erlang B distribution (Briley 1983, 151).

$$B(c,\mu) = \frac{\dfrac{\mu^c}{c!}}{\displaystyle\sum_{i=0}^{c} \frac{\mu^i}{i!}}$$

This involves only the mean value and the capacity. And while it looks pretty fancy, it is very easy to apply because the numerator is proportional to the Poisson value for c, given mean value μ, and the denominator is proportional to the cumulative Poisson value for c, given mean value μ, and in both cases the proportionality value is the same, so it cancels out.

Excel provides the built-in function Poisson (x, μ, cumulative true/false). If this last argument is false, then the function returns the Poisson probability, and if it is true, then the function returns the cumulative value. So, using Excel,

$$B(c,\mu) = \frac{Poisson(c,\mu,FALSE)}{Poisson(c,\mu,TRUE)}$$

Other spreadsheets may use slightly different nomenclature.

The Erlang B function gives the probability that the next customer will be denied immediate service and depends on two quantities: the average traffic level and the capacity.

In a hospital unit, the capacity is the number of beds. In a surgical unit, the capacity is the number of surgical teams or theaters. In an emergency department, the capacity is the number of doctors on duty.

The traffic, or demand, is the total number of treatment hours requested by all the patients who show up during the busy period, divided by the length, in hours, of the period of interest.

There are Web sites that do the Erlang B calculation, too, if spreadsheet calculations are not convenient. Try any Web search on 'Erlang B.'

THE ERLANG C DISTRIBUTION

Now consider the case where the patient who is not served immediately waits in queue. If the patient is willing to wait forever, eventually the patient will be served. So the measure of success is not whether or not the patient is served at all but rather whether the patient is served in a reasonable amount of time.

Erlang considered this as well, because it arises in telephony, too. How long will a telephone customer wait to hear "Number, please?" without blowing a gasket? Erlang's logic follows the Erlang B calculation, and assuming that readers will not be interested in the algebra, we will simply give the result.

The Erlang C distribution gives the likelihood that the next customer will be denied immediate service (but will be provided service at some later time). The formula is:

$$C(c,\mu) = \frac{\dfrac{\mu^c}{c!} + \dfrac{c}{c-\mu}}{\displaystyle\sum_{i=0}^{c-1}\dfrac{\mu^i}{i!} + \dfrac{\mu^c}{c!}\cdot\dfrac{c}{c-\mu}}$$

Happily, this doesn't have to be calculated by hand. There are commercial providers of Excel add-ins to do these and other calculations, and for the occasional user, there are Web sites that provide interactive, on the spot, free calculations (Koole 2002 or do a Web search; there are many others). Fill in the little on-screen template and get an immediate calculated answer.

Note that if c is quite close to μ, then both the numerator and the denominator go to infinity, so the result is indeterminate. What that means in practice is that there is no surge capacity to catch up if a lull in demand is followed by a surge in demand, even if the average traffic over the period does not exceed c. So, that won't work in the real world. To get any kind of performance at all, the capacity has to exceed the average traffic level for the period. Also, if the capacity is less than the average traffic level, the queue grows and grows without limit, so that won't work either.

So, Erlang C answers the important question, what is the likelihood that the next customer will be denied immediate service because others are already there, waiting in queue?

There is a related question: how many customers will have to wait very long in queue? That can be answered, too, provided one additional piece of information is provided, namely the average treatment time. The logical steps are these: What is the likelihood of a patient being added to the queue, and therefore what is the fraction of total traffic that is not served immediately and is therefore waiting in queue, and then what is the distribution in time of all that waiting?

Happily, the arithmetic is done for you by commercial software packages and by free Web sites (Koole 2002). The answer is given as a percentage of the total customer population required to wait more than a user-specific number of minutes (or hours or . . .).

Try this calculation and see. It's quite easy. Note that these Web sites will calculate any of the parameters given any sufficient combination of others. For instance, if the user specifies traffic level and the tolerable queuing service level, the computer will calculate the necessary capacity.

Appendix E
Emerging Technology—RFID

Six Sigma requires information. RFID is an enabling tech-nology that promises to supply information, economically, that has been lacking until now. Perhaps the biggest impact will be on patient cooperation and self-care.

WHAT IS IT?

RFID is short for *radio frequency identification*. It was created to replace the familiar bar code for product identification. Bar code has been around for 30 years and has slowly revolutionized the way inventory is kept, how cash registers work, and how drugs are tracked down to the single-dose level.

Healthcare was one of the slowest industries to adopt bar code beyond the shipping and receiving dock. Bar coding down to the single-dose level for drugs is still not universal despite the obvious improvement in information.

Bar code is now commonly, but not universally, used on patient ID wrist bands.

The disadvantage of bar code is that a line of sight is required between the scanner and the bar code tag. This makes bedside bar code clunky and ambulance application unworkable.

RFID consists of a tiny radio circuit and a tiny computer chip with memory. This is called the RFID tag. In the simplest case, the computer memory just holds a 'license plate number' that identifies the tag and therefore the item to which it is attached. There are universal product code rules for assigning the license plate number issued by the same industry groups that do the same for the traditional bar code.

The RFID tag is read by another radio that sends out a read-pulse. The tag absorbs enough energy from the read-pulse to have the strength to send back its license plate number. Thus the tag itself does not have to have its own energy source and therefore will work indefinitely, and there's nothing to wear out. The range at which this works depends on the strength of the read-pulse and the sensitivity of the read-receiver. It is generally in the several-inches range.

Longer ranges, up to football-field dimensions, are practical if the tag has a battery as a source of energy so that it can send back a strong signal. That is not practical for a can of beans on a store shelf, but it works fine today to inventory school buses in a huge parking lot.

The system is designed so that multiple tags do not interfere with each other, using the same concept as is used in Ethernet. The RFID industry standard calls for 800 tags to be read per second.

The tags are inherently read–write, although writing usually takes a stronger signal, which in practice means that writing is done at a shorter range.

Since this is all done with radio signals, line of sight is not required. The frequencies are those in the ISM (industry–science–medical) bands, of which there are several. Those commonly used are at 900 megahertz, 2.4 gigahertz, and 13.47 gigahertz.

Since the tags are read–write, the tags themselves can become a storehouse of information. For instance, routing instructions can be written into the tag so that warehouse transfer can be 'data driven' down to the case level.

The tags are too small to be noticed with the naked eye. Large ones are the size of a peppercorn. Since these are computer devices, they will only get smaller.

They are available today in all quantities and a wide range of capabilities. All major inventory/operations software suppliers are accommodating RFID.

MARKET ACCEPTANCE

Wal-Mart has ordered its top 100 suppliers to provide RFID on all cases and skids by January 2005, with extensive trials being done at this writing (2004). That comes to about a billion tags per year. All other Wal-Mart suppliers are lining up.

The Department of Defense has told its top 25,000 suppliers (!) to be on that same schedule.

Most major airlines have declared that they will use RFID tags on shipped luggage immediately. Some airports have this in service now.

The Japanese electronics industry, makers of tags, have projected a unit price of about a nickel within a few years. At this writing, unit prices are about a quarter.

When the unit price gets below a dime, the incentive is to put an RFID tag on every can of beans because the check-out cost and employee-related shrinkage goes down dramatically. No checker required. Scan the whole shopping basket at once.

HEALTHCARE DIRECT APPLICATIONS

The healthcare industry's purchasing agent association has specified that all suppliers will provide RFID tags, more or less on the Wal-Mart schedule. Same suppliers, so why not?

The major pharmaceutical companies have announced that they will provide RFID tags down to the single-dose level in the near future. Meanwhile, Purdue Pharma and Pfizer are shipping 100-pill bottles to pharmacies with RFID to the bottle level (Malykhina 2004, 20), starting with those that are subject to counterfeiting with the view that the RFID tags will complicate the life of the counterfeiter and protect patients from false drugs.

Success has already been shown with surgical sponges bearing RFID tags (Roebuck 2004). Sponges left in the patient can be read out even after the incision is closed, although it might be more timely to do the RFID check before the incision is closed. On the positive side, each sponge going in and each sponge coming out logs its unique license plate number, so the surgeon knows where to look for a sponge, if one is missing, before suturing.

At this writing, the National Institutes of Health is paying for a research project involving the University of Pittsburgh, MIT, and Massachusetts General Hospital to apply RFID tags on wristbands for patients taken into ambulances. This provides continuity in the identification of the patient and any medication or other actions during the ride. Traditional bar code is unworkable in this situation.

Boca Raton Community Hospital, Florida, is doing funded planning for the next hurricane crisis and is contemplating using RFID to track thousands of people through emergency care (Russell 2004).

While bedside application of RFID is not yet reported, it is an obvious application and much less demanding than ambulance RFID. This should do much to eliminate the clunkiness of bedside bar code.

RFID is being used in wristbands to identify surgical patients (Lok 2004, 25) at Jacobi Medical Center, the Bronx, and there are plans to build RFID into a new 500-bed facility there in the new year.

RFID has been approved by the FDA to mark the site for surgery (SurgiChip 2004).

RFID applies directly to building zone control. Hang an RFID reader on key doorframes and log who is going through. Flash a warning if the wrong person is going by. Use two RFID readers or a controllable antenna to get direction of movement. This requires that the person (or mobile equipment item) be tagged. Using this to control visitors would require that visitors be tagged. Most visitors wear a badge of some sort, and the RFID tag can be buried in the badge.

Keep track of wheelchairs? Keep track of infusion pumps? Mapping software has been used for years to keep track of over-the-road trucks, so mapping mobile equipment in a hospital is duck soup.

RFID tags can work with local readers, such as handheld devices, and they can work with area readers integrated into area wireless networks. The reader is a radio, not much different from the radios in wireless network nodes, wireless cards in PCs, and Bluetooth radios now common in computer peripheral devices. RFID is a key building block in the next round of improvements in patient safety, patient service, and productivity.

Appendix F
Sequential Testing Bases

A brief development of the statistics of sequential hypothesis testing.

CHECKLIST

☑ Permits the hypothesis to be tested after every sample, such as after every surgery.

☑ Useful in comparing local outcomes against national standards.

☑ Applies to testing a hypothesis against one alternative.

☑ Applies to any distributions, developed here for binomials.

☑ It's easy to do.

METHOD

It can be shown that the best method for testing a hypothesis against a single alternative is the likelihood-ratio test (Mood 1950, 365).

The objective is to determine on the basis of sequential tests whether the null hypothesis (that two distributions are the same) is supported or rejected to specified degrees of confidence against both false-negative and false-positive outcomes.

To apply the sequential method to binomial distributions, such as mortality from surgical procedures, the probability of success is needed for each of the two candidate distributions. For cases of interest here, those can be a national mortality rate and a local mortality rate. In addition, two parameters are required to assert the confidence levels against false-negative and false-positive outcomes.

It stands to reason that the higher the demand for confidence, the more sequential cases will be required. It also stands to reason that the closer the probabilities for the two distributions are to each other, the more sequential cases will be required to distinguish between the two.

Reasonable confidence levels are 90 percent.

Before starting the sequence, two limits will be computed from the confidence levels.

The upper limit, A, is computed by:

$$A \cong \frac{\text{Confidence level against false positives}}{\left(1 - \text{Confidence level against false negatives}\right)}$$

$$= \frac{90\%}{\left(100\% - 90\%\right)} = 9.0$$

The lower limit, B, is computed by:

$$B \cong \frac{\left(1 - \text{Confidence level against false positives}\right)}{\text{Confidence level against false negatives}}$$

$$= \frac{\left(100\% - 90\%\right)}{90\%} = 1/9 = 0.111$$

After each trial in the sequence, a *figure of merit* is calculated, according to the upcoming formula, and that figure of merit is compared to each of the limits A and B.

If the figure of merit exceeds A, then the null hypothesis is rejected. That means that the statistics support the assertion that the samples are being drawn from a distribution that is different from the reference distribution.

If the figure of merit is less than B, then the null hypothesis is accepted. That means that the statistics support the assertion that the samples are being drawn from a distribution that is the same as the reference distribution.

So, the sequence ends when either A or B is crossed. If A is crossed, the local mortality rate is different from the national mortality rate. If B is crossed, they are the same. Therefore, the objective is to cross B.

After each sequential case, say after case m, the ratio R_m is computed by:

$$R_m = \frac{\Pr(success, local)}{\Pr(success, national)} \text{ if successful, or}$$

$$R_m = \frac{\Pr(failure, local)}{\Pr(failure, national)} \text{ if not successful}$$

The figure of merit is the product of all the R_m values so far in the sequence.

$$Figure\ of\ merit = \prod_{i=1}^{m} R_i$$

Suppose the national success rate is 98.5 percent and that one fatality has occurred locally in 25 cases to date, giving an estimate for the local success rate of 24/25 = 96 percent. These can be used to calculate the R_m factors to apply sequentially as new cases are done and the outcomes observed.

$$R_m = \frac{\Pr(success, local)}{\Pr(success, national)} = \frac{96\%}{98.5\%} = 0.973 \text{ if successful, or}$$

$$R_m = \frac{\Pr(failure, local)}{\Pr(failure, national)} = \frac{4.0\%}{1.5\%} = 2.66 \text{ if not successful}$$

After the first case, the figure of merit will stand at either 0.973 or 2.66. After the second case, the figure of merit will be less, if that second case is successful, or greater, if that second case is not successful. And so on for subsequent cases.

SEQUENCES OF INTEREST

Here are possibilities:

1. The first few cases all fail. How many cases will be required to surpass limit A, which is 9.00, and show that the local distribution is distinct from the national distribution? Answer: the figure of merit grows by a factor of 2.66 each time, so after three cases the figure of merit will be greater than 9.00 and in fact will be 18.8. Therefore, three failures in the first three tries indicates that the local distribution is distinct from the national distribution.

2. The early cases are all successful. How many cases will be required to pass Limit B, which is 0.11, and show that the local distribution is the same as the national distribution? Answer: the figure of merit diminishes by a factor of 0.973 each time, so after 81 cases the figure of merit will be less than 0.111 and in fact will be 0.109. So, 81 successful cases out of the first 81 indicate that the local distribution is the same as the national distribution.

3. Suppose one case fails. How many more successful cases will be required to overcome this setback? It will take a total of 118 cases, one failing and 117 succeeding, which means that each failing case requires 36 successful cases (117–81) to overcome it.

4. Three failing cases at the beginning of the sequence mean failure of the project, as was stated above. But suppose a number of successful cases happen first, and then three failures transpire. How many early successful cases are required so that three successive failures do not mean failure of the project? Twenty-seven. Three successive adverse outcomes would certainly get attention for other reasons, though.

A graph illustrating the general characteristic of the figure of merit was shown on page 169 in Chapter 26. There it is seen that the figure of merit traces a gentle curve. If the same data were plotted on a ratio scale, the trace would be a straight line. Any spreadsheet will do this. The advantage of a straight line is that it is easy to extrapolate.

References

Abdelhak, M., ed. 2001. *Health Information: Management of a Strategic Resource*, 2nd ed. Philadelphia: Saunders Publishing.

Aguayo, R. 1990. *Dr. Deming, the American Who Taught the Japanese About Quality.* Secaucus, NJ: Lyle Stuart.

American Nurses Association (ANA). 2003. *Scope and Standards for Nurse Administrators,* 2nd ed. Washington, DC.

Aristotle. 1952. "Physics." *Britannica Great Books* 8. Chicago: University of Chicago Press: 259 et. seq.

Barry, R. F. 2003. *Nan: A Six Sigma Mystery.* Milwaukee: ASQ Quality Press.

———. 2004. *Nan's Arsonist: A Six Sigma Mystery.* Milwaukee: ASQ Quality Press.

Barry, R. F., A. C. Murcko, and C. E. Brubaker. 2002. *The Six Sigma Book for Healthcare.* Chicago: Health Administration Press.

Bellman, R. E. 1957. *Dynamic Programming.* Princeton University Press.

Blancett, S. S., and D. L. Flarey. 1998. *Health Care Outcomes: Collaborative, Path-Based Approaches.* Gaithersburg: Aspen.

Briley, B. E. 1983. *Introduction to Telephone Switching.* Reading, MA: Addison Wesley.

Burton, T. M. 2004. "Flop Factor: By Learning from Failures, Lilly Keeps Drug Pipeline Full." *Wall Street Journal* (April 21, 2004): 1 et seq.

Chicago Historical Society and the Trustees of Northwestern University. 1996. *The Great Conflagration.* www.chicagohs.org/fire/conflag.

Clark, K. 2004. "The Doctor Gets a Checkup, Firms Mean to Cut Medical Costs by 'Managing' Diseases." *U.S. News and World Report* (February 2, 2004): 44 et seq.

CMS. 2004. "CMS Urges States to Adopt Disease Management Programs, Agency Will Match State Costs." CMS Office of Public Affairs, Centers for Medicare and Medicaid Services. (February 26, 2004.) www.cms.hhs.gov/media/press/release.asp?Counter=967.

Flarey, D. L., and S. S. Blancett. 1998. *Cardiovascular Outcomes: Collaborative, Path-Based Approaches.* Gaithersburg: Aspen.

Friedman, M. B. 2004. Pittsburgh, PA: AugmenTech, Inc. Personal communication.

Gee, E. P. 2004. *Service Line Success: Eight Essential Rules.* Chicago: ACHE Health Administration Press.

Gerteis, M., ed. 1993. *Through the Patient's Eyes: Understanding and Promoting Patient-Centered Care.* San Francisco: Jossey-Bass.

HHS. 1998. Centers for Disease Prevention and Control. DHHS (NIOHS) Publication 97–111. Atlanta: National Institute for Occupational Health and Safety.

JCAHO. 2004. *Hospital Accreditation Standards.* Chicago: Joint Commission on Accreditation of Healthcare Organizations.

JNCCN. 2004. "Clinical Practice Guidelines in Oncology, Cervical Cancer." *Journal of the National Comprehensive Cancer Network* 2, no. 6 (November 2004).

Juran, J. M. 1995. *Managerial Breakthrough,* revised edition. New York: McGraw-Hill.

Koole, G., and M. Bijvank. 2002. "Erlang-C Calculator," Vrije Universiteit van Amsterdam. www.cs.vu.nl/~koole/ccmath/ErlangC.php. (In English).

KPMG. 2002. What Patients Really Think of the New Health Network (UK). www.newhealthnetwork.co.uk/Documents/Publication/public_nhs_survey.pdf. (February 2002).

Landro, L. 2003. "Six Prescriptions to Ease Rationing in U.S. Healthcare." *Wall Street Journal* (December 22, 2003).

Leveson, N. G. 1995. *Safeware: System Safety and Computers.* New York: Addison Wesley.

Liker, J. K. 2004. *The Toyota Way: 14 Management Rules from the World's Greatest Manufacturing Company.* New York: McGraw-Hill. Rule 14.

Llewellyn, A., and K. Moreo. 2001. *Case Management Review & Resource Manual: The Essence of Case Management.* Washington:

Institute for Research, Education, and Consultation at the American Nurses Credentialing Center.

Lok, C. 2004. "Wrist Radio Tags." *Technology Review Magazine* (November 2004).

Malykhina, E. 2004. "Drugmaker Ships RFID Tags with OxyContin." *Information Week* (November 22, 2004): 20.

Mercer, J., and H. Arlen. 1944. *Ac-cen-tchu-ate the Positive.* Harwin Music Co.

NYAM. 2000. New York Academy of Medicine Web site http://www.ebmny.org/ which is sponsored by the New York Academy of Medicine in partnership with the Evidence-Based Medicine Committee of the American College of Physicians, New York Chapter with financial support from the National Institutes of Health.

NYU Medical Center. 2004. *Patient Handouts: Patient Pathways.* NYU Medical Center, Patient and Family Education. library.med.nyu.edu/HCC/handouts/pathway.html.

Pande, P. S., R. P. Neuman, and R. R. Cavanaugh. 2000. *The Six Sigma Way.* New York: McGraw-Hill: 54.

Pittsburgh Regional Healthcare Initiative (PRHI). 2004. Quarterly newsletter. Pittsburgh, PA: PRHI. www.prhi.org.

Reh, F. J. 2002. *Pareto's Principle: The 80/20 Rule.* management.about.com/cs/generalmanagement/a/Pareto081202.htm.

Roebuck, K. 2004. "Surgical Tracking Device Soaks Up Top Honors." *Pittsburgh Tribune Review* (March 30, 2004).

Russell, M. 2004. Boca Raton, FL: Boca Raton Community Hospital. Personal communication. December 1.

Smith, A. 1776. *Wealth of Nations.* First published in 1776, available in many editions.

State University of Iowa. 2004. *Evidence Based Nursing Practice.* www.nursing.uiowa.edu/sites/users/gardery/ebp/protocols.htm.

SurgiChip. 2004. "Identification Tag to Mark Sites Where a Patient Will Have Surgery," Palm Beach Gardens, Florida: SurgiChip. Company press release on Web site www.surgichip.com.

Taguchi, G., S. Chowdhury, and S. Taguchi. 1999. *Robust Engineering.* New York: McGraw-Hill.

Tucker, A. L., and A. C. Edmondson. 2003. "Why Hospitals Don't Learn from Failures: Organizational and Psychological Dynamics That Inhibit System Change." *California Management Review* 45, no. 2 (Winter 2003).

Weinberg, D. B. 2003. *Code Green*. Ithaca: Cornell University Press.

Wojner, A. W. 2001. *Outcomes Management. Applications to Clinical Practice*. St. Louis: Mosby.

Wysocki, B., Jr. 2004. "To Fix Health Care, Hospitals Take Tips from Factory Floor. Adopting Toyota Techniques Can Cut Costs, Wait Times; Ferreting Out an Infection. What Paul O'Neill's Been Up To." *Wall Street Journal* CCXLIII, no. 70 (April 09, 2004): 1, 6.

Index